Autologous Techniques to Fill Bone Defects for Acute Fractures and Nonunions

Guest Editors

HANS C. PAPE, MD, FACS
TIMOTHY G. WEBER, MD

ORTHOPEDIC CLINICS OF NORTH AMERICA

www.orthopedic.theclinics.com

January 2010 • Volume 41 • Number 1

SAUNDERS an imprint of ELSEVIER, Inc.

W.B. SAUNDERS COMPANY
A Division of Elsevier Inc.

1600 John F. Kennedy Blvd. • Suite 1800 • Philadelphia, PA 19103-2899.

http://www.orthopedic.theclinics.com

ORTHOPEDIC CLINICS OF NORTH AMERICA Volume 41, Number 1
January 2010 ISSN 0030-5898, ISBN-13: 978-1-4377-1847-8

Editor: Debora Dellapena
Developmental Editor: Donald Mumford

Orthopedic Clinics of North America (ISSN 0030-5898) is published quarterly by Elsevier Inc., 360 Park Avenue South, New York, NY 10010-1710. Months of issue are January, April, July, and October. Business and Editorial Offices: 1600 John F. Kennedy Blvd., Suite 1800, Philadelphia, PA 19103-2899. Customer Service Office: 3251 Riverport Lane, Maryland Heights, MO 63043. Periodicals postage paid at New York, NY and additional mailing offices. Subscription prices are $251.00 per year for (US individuals), $458.00 per year for (US institutions), $297.00 per year (Canadian individuals), $549.00 per year (Canadian institutions), $366.00 per year (international individuals), $549.00 per year (international institutions), $126.00 per year (US students), $182.00 per year (Canadian and international students). Foreign air speed delivery is included in all *Clinics* subscription prices. All prices are subject to change without notice. **POSTMASTER:** Send address changes to *Orthopedic Clinics of North America*, Elsevier Periodicals Customer Service, 3251 Riverport Lane, Maryland Heights, MO 63043. Customer Service (orders, claims, online, change of address): Elsevier Periodicals Customer Service, 11830 Westline Industrial Drive, St. Louis, MO 63146. Tel: 1-800-654-2452 (U.S. and Canada); 314-447-8871 (outside U.S. and Canada). Fax: 314-447-8024. E-mail: journalscustomerservice-usa@elsevier.com (for print support); journalsonlinesupport-usa@elsevier.com (for online support).

Reprints. For copies of 100 or more, of articles in this publication, please contact the Commercial Reprints Department, Elsevier Inc., 360 Park Avenue South, New York, NY 10010-1710. Tel.: 212-633-3812; Fax: 212-462-1935; Email: reprints@elsevier.com.

Orthopedic Clinics of North America is covered in *MEDLINE/PubMed (Index Medicus)*, Cinahl, Excerpta Medica, and *Cumulative Index to Nursing and Allied Health Literature*.

Printed in the United States of America

Transferred to Digital Printing, 2011

Contributors

GUEST EDITORS

HANS C. PAPE, MD, FACS
W. Pauwels Professor and Chairman,
Department of Orthopedics and Trauma,
University of Aachen Medical Center,
Aachen, Germany

TIMOTHY G. WEBER, MD
Traumatologist, OrthoIndy, Indianapolis,
Indiana

AUTHORS

FANI ANAGNOSTOU, DM
Laboratoire de Bioingénierie et Biomécanique
Ostéo-articulaires, Université
Paris-Diderot, Paris, France

THIERRY BEGUE, MD
Orthopedic Surgeon, Department of
Orthopedics and Traumatology, Avicenne
Hospital, Medical University of Paris, Bobigny,
France

MORAD BENSIDHOUM, PhD
Laboratoire de Bioingénierie et Biomécanique
Ostéo-articulaires, Université
Paris-Diderot, Paris, France

DAVID S. BROKAW, MD
OrthoIndy, Indianapolis, Indiana

LISA K. CANNADA, MD
Associate Professor, Department of
Orthopedic Surgery, St Louis University, St
Louis, Missouri

JANET D. CONWAY, MD
Head of Bone and Joint Infection, International
Center for Limb Lengthening, Rubin Institute
for Advanced Orthopedics, Sinai Hospital of
Baltimore, Baltimore, Maryland

HARALAMPOS T. DINOPOULOS, MD
Trauma Fellow, Academic Department
of Trauma and Orthopedic Surgery, University
of Leeds, Leeds, United Kingdom

CHRISTOPHER G. FINKEMEIER, MD, MBA
Co-director, Orthopedic Trauma Surgeons
of Northern California, Sutter Roseville
Medical Center, Roseville, California

**PETER V. GIANNOUDIS, BSc, MB, MD,
FRCS**
Professor, Department of Trauma and
Orthopedic Surgery, University of Leeds,
United Kingdom; Professor, Academic
Orthopedic Unit, Leeds General Infirmary
University Hospital, Leeds, United Kingdom

JAMES M. GREEN, BS
Synthes, Paoli, Pennsylvania

GENEVIÈVE GUILLEMIN, PhD
Laboratoire de Bioingénierie et
Biomécanique Ostéo-articulaires,
Université Paris-Diderot, Paris, France

DAVID J. HAK, MD, MBA
Associate Professor, Department of
Orthopedic Surgery, Denver Health
University of Colorado, Denver, Colorado

DOMINGO HALLARE, MD
Director, Orthopedic Trauma, Department
of Orthopedics, Kaiser Permanente
South Sacramento, Sacramento, California

DIDIER HANNOUCHE, DM, PhD
Service de Chirurgie Orthopédique, Hôpital
Lariboisière, Paris, France

BRADLEY A. JELEN, DO
OrthoIndy, Indianapolis, Indiana

DEAN C. MAAR, MD
OrthoIndy, Indianapolis, Indiana

JAMES T. MARINO, MD
Resident, Department of Orthopedic Surgery,
Atlanta Medical Center, Atlanta, Georgia

ALAIN C. MASQUELET, MD
Department Head of Orthopedics and Trauma,
Orthopedic Surgeon, Avicenne Hospital,
Medical University of Paris, Bobigny, France

JEFFREY W. MAST, MD
Associate Clinical Professor, University of
Nevada Reno, Mammoth Orthopedics and
Sports Medicine, Sierra Park Orthopedics,
Mammoth Lakes, California

TODD A. McCALL, MD
Orthopaedic Clinics of Daytona Beach,
Daytona Beach, Florida

RICHARD P. MEINIG, MD
Department of Orthopedics, Front Range
Orthopedic Association, Memorial Hospital,
Colorado Springs, Colorado

FARIBA MOEINPOUR, MS
Research Assistant, Center for Surgical
Research, The University of Alabama at
Birmingham, Birmingham, Alabama

DANA MUSAPATIKA, MS, MSc
Synthes, Paoli, Pennsylvania

RAFAEL NEIMAN, MD
Co-director, Orthopedic Trauma Surgeons
of Northern California, Sutter Roseville Medical
Center, Roseville, California

HANS C. PAPE, MD, FACS
W. Pauwels Professor and Chairman,
Department of Orthopedics and Trauma,
University of Aachen Medical Center,
Aachen, Germany

PHILIPPE PÉLISSIER, DM
Service de Chirurgie Plastique, Groupe
Hospitalier Pellegrin, Bordeaux, France

JOHN J. PERRY, MD
Associate Clinical Professor, University
of Nevada Reno, Mammoth Orthopedics
and Sports Medicine, Mammoth Lakes,
California

HERVÉ PETITE, PhD
Laboratoire de Bioingénierie et Biomécanique
Ostéo-articulaires, Université
Paris-Diderot, Paris, France

JASON L. PITTMAN, MD, PhD
Resident, Department of Surgery, University of
Colorado, Aurora, Colorado

ASHOKE K. SATHY, MD
Assistant Professor, Department of
Orthopedics, The University of Alabama at
Birmingham, Birmingham, Alabama

ANGELA V. SCHARFENBERGER, MD
University Orthopedic Consultants,
Edmonton, Alberta, Canada

D. KEVIN SCHEID, MD
OrthoIndy, Indianapolis, Indiana

MELANIE R. SHIPPS, BS
OrthoIndy, Indianapolis, Indiana

PETER A. SISKA, MD
Assistant Professor, University of Pittsburgh,
Pittsburgh, Pennsylvania

JAMES P. STANNARD, MD
J. Vernon Luck Sr Distinguished Professor
and Chairman, Department of Orthopedics,
University of Alabama at Birmingham,
Birmingham, Alabama

RENA L. STEWART, MD
Assistant Professor, Department of
Orthopedics, Division of Orthopedics Trauma,
The University of Alabama at Birmingham,
Birmingham, Alabama

MARCUS B. STONE, PhD
Alegius Consulting, Avon, Indiana

IVAN S. TARKIN, MD
Assistant Professor, Department of Orthopedic
Surgery, Division of Traumatology, Interim
Chief Orthopedic Traumatology, University of
Pittsburgh, Pittsburgh, Pennsylvania

VÉRONIQUE VIATEAU, DMV, PhD
Unité Pédagogique de Pathologie
Chirurgicale, Ecole Nationale Vétérinaire
d'Alfort, Maisons-Alfort, France

DAVID A. VOLGAS, MD
Associate Professor, Department of
Orthopedics, Division of Orthopedics
Trauma, The University of Alabama
at Birmingham, Birmingham,
Alabama

TIMOTHY G. WEBER, MD
Traumatologist, OrthoIndy, Indianapolis,
Indiana

ANDREA WIESE, MD
Department of Orthopedic Trauma, RWTH
Aachen University Medical Center, Aachen,
Germany

BRENT WINTER, MD
West Valley City, Utah

BORIS A. ZELLE, MD
University of Pittsburgh, Pittsburgh,
Pennsylvania

BRUCE H. ZIRAN, MD
Director of Orthopedic Trauma, Department
of Orthopedic Surgery, Atlanta Medical Center,
Atlanta, Georgia

Contents

Bone defects represent a difficult problem for the clinician. They entail a sustained increase in hospitalization, risk of complications, and associated increase in expenses. This article discusses bone defects caused by high-energy injuries, bone loss, infected nonunions, and nonunions.

The healing of fractures and nonunions has significant science background to it; however, the application of the products in the surgeon's hands should be considered an art in the science of bone healing. The surgeon must choose adequate fixation for stability and to promote healing by not making the construct too stiff. If a bone graft substitute is necessary, the surgeon must choose the type of bone graft substitute depending on patient factors and surgeon factors involving the treatment of the fracture.

Bone is the second most commonly implanted material in the human body, after blood transfusion, with an estimated 600,000 grafts performed annually. Although the market for bone graft substitutes is more than $1 billion, that of bone graft itself is still more than half that amount. Reports of autologous bone grafting date back to the ancient Egyptians, yet the modern scientific study of grafting began in the early 19th century. Since then, the indications, methodology, and science of bone grafts in nonunion and bone loss have been established and refined, and new methods of harvesting and treatment are being developed and implemented. This article describes the use of solid and cancellous bone graft in the treatment of acute bone loss and nonunion.

Clinical, experimental, and fundamental studies have shown the interest of a foreign body-induced membrane to promote the consolidation of a conventional cancellous bone autograft for reconstruction of long bone defects. The main properties of the membrane are to prevent the resorption of the graft and to secrete growth factors. The induced membrane appears as a biological chamber, which allows the conception of numerous experimental models of bone reconstruction. This concept could probably be extended to other tissue repair.

The reconstruction of large bone defects remains a clinically challenging condition. Although many treatment approaches exist, they all have limitations. Recently, bioresorbable polylactide membranes have become commercially available. These membranes, when applied to bone defects, enhance bone healing by direct osteoconduction, exclusion of nonosseous tissues, and enhancing the osteogenic environment for autologous grafts. When combined with appropriate internal fixation and autologous bone graft, bioresorbable polylactide membranes allow for single-step reconstruction of large bone defects.

Animal experiments using the induced membrane procedure for bone tissue engineering purposes have provided evidence that the membrane has structural characteristics and biologic properties that may be used for bone tissue engineering purposes. Clinically relevant animal models have demonstrated that standardized particulate bone constructs can be used to repair large bone defects using the procedure and that the osteogenic ability of these constructs partially approaches that of bone autografts.

Bone harvested by intramedullary reaming offers a minimally invasive alternative to harvesting bone from the iliac crest, which has long been considered the gold standard for autogenous bone grafting. The biologic potential of intramedullary reaming material has been studied both in vitro and in vivo. The material provides osteogenic, osteoinductive, and osteoconductive properties that are comparable to the material harvested from the iliac crest. In addition to the ability to obtain a large volume of bone, the graft harvested by the Reamer-Irrigator-Aspirator has been shown to be rich in growth factors, including BMP-2, TGF-β1, IGF-I, FGFa, and PDGFbb.

Treatment of large segmental defects using conventional autogenous iliac crest bone graft can be limited by volume of cancellous bone and donor site morbidity. The reamer-irrigator-aspirator (RIA) technique allows access to a large volume of cancellous bone graft containing growth factors with potency equal to or greater than autograft material from the iliac crest. The purpose of this study was to evaluate the effectiveness of RIA-harvested autogenous bone graft for treating large segmental defects of long bones.

Revision surgery of the proximal femur with bone loss secondary to failed cephalo-medullary nails is problematic and becoming more prevalent as their use grows. This article presents a technique of deformity correction, bone graft techniques that reconstitute residual defects, and definitive fixation using load-sharing devices that provide immediate stability for bone healing and early rehabilitation. Preoperative planning and the potential advantages and disadvantages of newer fixed-angled plates versus established implants are discussed. With proper planning, surgical execution with proved techniques, augmented by the addition of newer graft harvesting techniques, anatomic restoration, and bone reconstitution with healing, has invariably been the result.

A thoughtful treatment algorithm is required to optimally treat distal tibia nonunion. A healthy respect for the tenuous soft tissue envelope, compromised vascularity, and challenging mechanical environment is advisable. Achieving osseous union and improved functionality requires an individualized plan of care based on the personality of the nonunion and host. Attention must be focused on providing mechanical stability at the site of nonunion and providing biologic supplementation.

Orthopedic Clinics of North America

THE CLINICS ARE NOW AVAILABLE ONLINE!

Access your subscription at:
www.theclinics.com

Preface

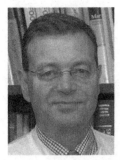 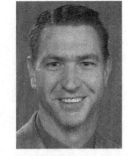

Hans C. Pape, MD, FACS   Timothy G. Weber, MD
Guest Editors

The management of traumatic bone defect continues to be a tremendous challenge to orthopedic trauma surgeons. Although many products that stimulate the growth of bone and replace defects have become available within the past decades, autologous bone continues to have ideal biologic properties. Although some of the well-described techniques to grow bone, such as distraction osteogenesis, have incurrent risks of infections, newer methods have become available to treat bone defects in the presence of an infection.

These techniques are well illustrated in this issue of *Orthopedic Clinics of North America*. The clinical reports and the basic science information illustrate the vast clinical experience of the authors of this issue.

As guest editors we would like to thank the authors for their excellent contributions and their outstanding service to make this another highlight issue. It has been a great honor to have had the opportunity to serve as guest editors of *Orthopedic Clinics of North America*. We would like to express our special thanks to Jim Green, who has helped to put this issue together, and to Mrs Deb Dellapena for continuous effort and help.

Hans C. Pape, MD, FACS
Department of Orthopedics/Trauma
University of Aachen Medical Center
30 Pauwels Street
Aachen 52074, Germany

Timothy G. Weber, MD
OrthoIndy, 1801 North Senate Boulevard, # 200
Indianapolis, IN 46202, USA

E-mail addresses:
papehc@aol.com (H.C. Pape)
tgweber@orthoindy.com (T.G. Weber)

Orthop Clin N Am 41 (2010) xiii
doi:10.1016/j.ocl.2009.09.001
0030-5898/09/$ – see front matter

Bone Defects Caused by High-energy Injuries, Bone Loss, Infected Nonunions, and Nonunions

Andrea Wiese, MD[a,b], Hans C. Pape, MD, FACS[c,*]

KEYWORDS
- Trauma • Bone loss • Operations • Technical tricks
- Femur fractures

Bone defects represent a difficult problem for the clinician. They entail a sustained increase in hospitalization, risk of complications, and associated increase in expenses (**Fig. 1**). The average cost for patients suffering from fractures following motor vehicle accidents has been estimated at US$10,000 per case.[1,2] Nonunions cost about US$25,000; the estimate varies according to the location of the fracture site (humerus<tibia< femur).[3] These direct costs apply only to nonunions that heal uneventfully after the first revision surgery. In contrast, bone loss imposes a longer period of treatment, and has an even higher complication rate and associated costs. To our knowledge, there is no published information on the costs incurred as a result of bone loss.

The term bone loss may refer either to structural defects and regions of missing bone caused by external factors or true defects and structural loss within existing bone, such as in osteopenia. **Fig. 2** gives an overview of causes for bone loss.

By definition, primary and secondary bone loss can be differentiated. Primary bone loss may occur in bone diseases, such as malignancy. Secondary bone loss is most commonly caused by metastatic disease. Tumor metastases may have either osteoblastic or osteolytic features. Both damage the bone in terms of structure, nutrition, and metabolism. Trauma is the most common cause of bone defects (**Fig. 3**).

In the planning of treatment for bone loss, several factors must be considered: the quality of the soft tissue envelope, the quality of vascular supply, and the presence or absence of an infection. In terms of treatment there is a wide variety of options.

In the acute setting, shortening of the bone may be considered, as depicted in **Fig. 4**. If shortening is considered, several concepts have to be considered. First, the bony ends should be adapted to allow the best contact possible. Second, the viability of the bone is of pivotal importance, thus requiring planned revision surgery. Third, coverage of all bony structures is crucial to avoid infection. In humeral and tibial defects this may be used if the distance between the fracture ends ranges up to 2 inches. In the femur, larger defects may be treated using this technique. According to isolated reports, defects of up to 3 inches have been treated by shortening.[4,5] The advantage of acute shortening is that there is

[a] Department of Orthopedic Trauma, Aachen University Medical Center, Pauwelsstr. 30, Aachen 52074, Germany
[b] Department of Orthopedic Surgery, University of Aachen Medical Center, Pauwelsstr. 30, Aachen 52074, Germany
[c] Department of Orthopedics, University of Pittsburgh Medical Center, 3471 Fifth Avenue, Pittsburgh, PA 15217, USA
* Corresponding author.
E-mail address: papehc@upmc.edu (H.C. Pape).

Orthop Clin N Am 41 (2010) 1–4
doi:10.1016/j.ocl.2009.07.003
0030-5898/09/$ – see front matter © 2010 Elsevier Inc. All rights reserved.

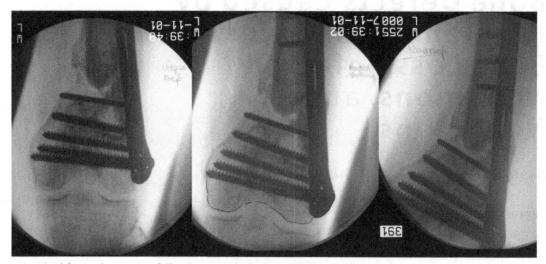

Fig. 1. Distal femoral nonunion following a nonlocked lateral plate osteosynthesis.

a greater chance of avoiding the necessity of free flap coverage by facilitating secondary definitive closure or early skin grafting. Disadvantages of this approach include shortening of the affected limb and prolonged treatment until the preinjury length is achieved.

Other treatment options for bone loss are autologous bone grafting, heterologous bone grafting, or the use of bone matrices to fill the void.[6] The latter may be combined with growth factors, osteogenic cells, or both. Although these techniques may be promising tools for the future, currently the number of clinical studies determining their usefulness is limited.[7]

Autologous bone continues to have optimal properties for adequate growth; however, the morbidity after iliac crest bone grafting is considerable[8] and therefore its status as the gold standard for filling bone defects has been questioned. The availability of autologous bone graft continues to be an issue. Although one may argue that multiple sites can be used, such as the elbow, the tibial plateau, and the posterior superior iliac spine, donor site morbidity continues to be a problem and has decreased the options for autologous grafting.

To overcome this drawback, Pelissier and colleagues described a new technique. Temporary filling of the gap with bone cement induces the development of a well vascularized membrane. This membrane appears to have an extraordinary capacity to nourish the grafted material. In their case series of large bone grafts, the main indication is chronic infection that has been treated with aggressive debridement and bone resection.[9] The issue of what is the maximum volume that can be generated from a certain graft site must still be resolved for this technique.

One solution may lie in the use of the reamer irrigator aspirator (RIA). This new technique addresses the issues of limited volume by using the femoral canal and the femoral condyles as sources of cancellous bone. It generates a large volume of bone graft that is harvested as a jolt material. The

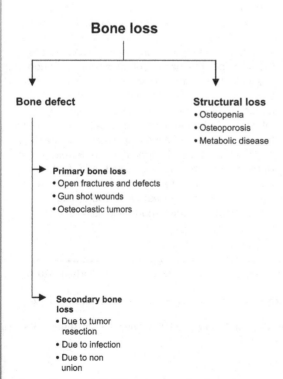

Fig. 2. Overview of different causes for bone loss.

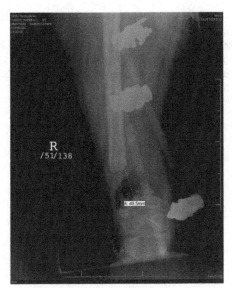

Fig. 3. Large osseous defect following posttraumatic osteonecrosis. This resulted in a secondary resection of 2 inches of the distal femur.

surface of this jolt bone graft is enlarged and has excellent molding capacities. Moreover, a large volume of cancellous bone can be harvested.[10] The jolt material obtained has been proven to have excellent osteogenic properties and allows for the filling of large defects. Moreover, it appears that pelvic pain is avoided and there appears to be no particular pain in the area of the incision.

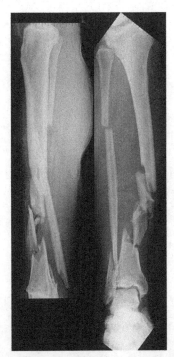

Fig. 4. Bone loss in an OIII b open tibia fracture.

As in the case of Pelissier's technique, a large series has not yet been published to date; however, it seems to be in widespread use even in the absence of level I or II evidence. Many case reports and smaller series reinforce the fact that clinicians have been convinced about the effectiveness and usefulness of the method.[10]

Although the Pelissier technique has been described specifically for complicated situations such as bone loss for infected nonunions, the uses of the RIA technique appear to differ in this scenario. In infected nonunions its benefit appears to lie not so much in its ability to provide new bone, but in its cleansing effects caused by the continuous rinsing of the medullary canal. Regardless of these new techniques, situations difficult to resolve continue to occur.

Currently there is no universally accepted algorithm that describes how to treat bone defects. To date, the surgeon often must decide on a case-by-case basis. The quality of the soft tissues, local perfusion, availability of vascular supply for possible flap coverage, and other factors must be reconsidered each time a bone loss is treated. Hopefully this issue will provide more insight about when the use of autologous bone graft is indicated, and when other techniques or substitutes should be administered instead.

REFERENCES

1. Maraste P, Persson U, Berntman M. Long-term follow-up and consequences for severe road traffic injuries—treatment costs and health impairment in Sweden in the 1960s and the 1990s. Health Policy 2003;66(2):147–58.
2. Corso P, Finkelstein E, Miller T, et al. Incidence and lifetime costs of injuries in the United States. Inj Prev 2006;12(4):212–8.
3. Donaldson LH, Brooke K, Faux SG. Orthopaedic trauma from road crashes: is enough being done? Aust Health Rev 2009;33(1):72–83.
4. Mahaluxmivala J, Nadarajah R, Allen PW, et al. Ilizarov external fixator: acute shortening and lengthening versus bone transport in the management of tibial non-unions. Injury 2005; 36:662–8.
5. Watson JT. Treatment of tibial fractures with bone loss. Tech Orthop 1996;11:132–43.
6. Maurer SG, Baitner AC, Di Cesare PE. Reconstruction of the failed femoral component and proximal femoral bone loss in revision hip surgery. J Am Acad Orthop Surg 2000;8:354–63.
7. Cancedda R, Giannoni P, Mastrogiacomo M. A tissue engineering approach to bone repair in large animal models and in clinical practice. Biomaterials 2007;28(29):4240–50.

8. Yajima H, Tamai S, Mizumoto S, et al. Vascularized fibular grafts in the treatment of ostemyelitis and infected non-union. Clin Orthop 1993;293:256–64.

9. Pelissier PH, Masquelet AC, Bareille R, et al. Induced membranes secrete growth factors including vascular and osteoinductive factors and could stimulate bone regeneration. J Orthop Res 2004;22(1):73–9.

10. Kobbe P, Tarkin IS, Pape HC. Use of the 'reamer irrigator aspirator' system for non-infected tibial non-union after failed iliac crest grafting. Injury 2008; 39:796–800.

Viable Bone and Circulatory Factors Required for Survival of Bone Grafts

Lisa K. Cannada, MD

KEYWORDS

- Non-union • Autograft • Demineralized bone matrix
- Bone morphogenetic proteins
- Platelet derived growth factor • Fracture

Bone grafts and bone graft substitutes are necessary in trauma surgery for a variety of reasons. Acutely, there are various bone grafts and substitutes used in fracture fixation to provide scaffolding for periarticular fracture fixation. Subacute use of bone grafts and substitutes occurs when the fracture does not heal. When fractures fail to progress in healing, each case needs to be evaluated as to why fracture healing did not occur.

Let's first look at what happens when a fracture occurs. The blood supply in bone comes from three sources: the intramedullary artery, periosteal vessels, and metaphyseal vessels. The injury itself disrupts some of the blood supply. The more severe the soft tissue injury accompanying the fracture, the more severe the disruption of the blood supply. With fracture fixation, the blood supply is disrupted during surgery by stripping the periosteal vessels with plate fixation or reaming with intramedullary nail placement. Recently, fracture fixation has become more biologically friendly attempting to preserve the periosteal vessels as much as can be possible. In addition to the vessels, the surrounding soft tissue envelope is just as important.

With a fracture, there is the release of numerous growth factors to induce the healing process.[1–3] There are mesenchymal stem cells found in the bone marrow, the periosteum, and soft tissue and they differentiate into chondrogenic and osteogenic cells.[2] Osteoblasts form bone directly to the intramembranous ossification, chondroblasts begin to form soft callous, and bone is formed through endochondral ossification. These processes are under the influence of many growth factors including platelet-derived growth factor (PDGF) and vascular endothelial growth factor (VEGF) transforming growth factor (TGF)-beta.[1] The vascular supplies are very important for the formation of bone. It is necessary throughout the healing process for the healing to occur, including with nonunions.

The fracture hematoma that is present affects the oxygen tension of the tissues and it is the oxygen tension that has a role in the type of healing along with the fracture stability with the fracture treatment. Osteoprogenitor cells proliferate in areas of increased oxygen tension and decreased strength, so that when you have an area of high oxygen tension and no strain, you get formation of woven bone directly.[3] In regions of intermediate strain and low oxygen tension you have a different environment and callous formation occurs.[3] A fibrocartilaginous callous bridges across the fracture site. The cartilage then can reduce the strain and lead to bone formation.

The stability imparted by the fixation chosen also influences healing. Primary bone healing occurs with rigid stability and secondary healing happens with relative stability. Primary healing has apposition of fracture ends when there is bone-on-bone

Disclosure: The author previously was a consultant for Medtronic Sofamer Danek.
Department of Orthopedic Surgery, St Louis University, 3635 Vista Avenue, 7th floor, St Louis, MO 63110, USA
E-mail address: Lcannada@slu.edu

Orthop Clin N Am 41 (2010) 5–13
doi:10.1016/j.ocl.2009.07.008

contact. Cutting cones cross the fracture, the osteoclasts create a tunnel, and the osteoblasts fill in the tunnel. New Haversion systems provide a pathway for blood vessels. The stiffness and strength of this construct increase as osteoblasts form new bone. With secondary fracture healing, you get healing with a callus. The vascular response varies according to the oxygen tension on the tissues just discussed and the mechanical stability. If you have an area where there is continued strain, that can be difficult to form bone and you may be more likely to get a fibrous nonunion.

Patient factors that affect bone healing include the use of nicotine.[3–6] Nicotine affects the oxygen environment, thus giving you a low oxygen environment, and you are more likely to have fibrous tissue form and the healing process can take longer or the fracture may not heal at all. Medications that the patient takes affect the healing process. Nonsteroidal anti-inflammatory agents affect bone healing by disrupting the inflammatory cycle, which occurs early in fracture healing.[3,4] Patients with diabetes have delayed healing and, in addition, they may have additional nutritional factors that affect their healing.[3–6] Brinker and colleagues[7] found a high percentage of male patients treated for nonunion had a nutritional abnormality. Most importantly, the patient's soft tissue injury is key in promoting fracture healing. Gaston and colleagues[8] evaluated tibia fractures and found that the most significantly affected fracture healing was the soft tissue injury. The soft tissue envelope is not to be taken lightly and disruptions in handling the soft tissues can affect the healing process. Likewise, when a nonunion occurs, it is important to create the environment to allow healing to begin to occur.

In order for bone healing to occur, you need an adequate blood supply and adequate mechanical stability. There are different three types of nonunions. Atrophic nonunions do not have adequate biology for healing. Oligotrophic and hypertrophic nonunions are nonunions that have callous formation present and are making attempts to heal[9]; however, the union is fibrous tissue and the fracture needs stability to promote healing. With any nonunion it is important to rule out infection as a cause. Preoperative laboratory values should be obtained including erythrocyte sedimentation rate (ESR), C reactive protein (CRP), and complete blood count (CBC) with differential.[6] Further radiographic studies may be helpful if infection is suspected.

Once the nonunion is diagnosed, planning begins to promote healing. Further surgery is often necessary and may involve bone grafting. The choice of whether to use autograft or a bone graft substitute must be made. Bone graft substitutes represent a \$2.5 billion industry.[10] No matter what type of bone graft is chosen, there must be a conducive environment, biologically and mechanically, to promote healing.

It is important to understand the terminology of bone grafting. Osteoconductive bone grafts are those that provide scaffolding for new bone growth. New bone growth occurs by creeping substitution. This is a more passive response. Osteoinductive bone graft substitutes form bone in a more active process. Anything classified as osteoinductive will induce new bone formation where bone would not normally form.[5] An osteogenic bone graft involves generation of bone directly from bone-forming cells.

No matter what product is chosen, the ultimate goal is fracture healing. No one product represents a magic potion to promote healing. The product chosen must be right for the environment and mechanical stability of the fracture.

MECHANICAL STABILITY

The importance of mechanical stability on healing is known. Bone healing is an active process and stability plays a key role in this process. Bone formation is a continuous process and initiates early on in embryogenesis and continues throughout life. Bone remodeling after fracture continues in response to the stresses that are placed on it. When a fracture occurs, some heal with callus in which there was some motion or, with primary bone healing, no callous formation occurs.

Le and colleagues[11] looked at which changes in the signaling process cause cartilage or bony callous. The authors wanted to evaluate the mechanism in which mesenchymal stem cells (MSC) sense the disparities between a stable and unstable fracture environment and how the healing occurs. The authors found that Indian hedgehog (IHH), which regulates the aspects of chondrocyte maturation during early fetal and early postnatal bone development, was expressed earlier in a non-stabilized fracture model as compared with those with a stabilized fracture.[11] IHH exerts its effect on chondrocyte maturation through feedback involving bone morphogenetic proteins and transcription factors.[11] Stabilizing the fracture decreases or minimizes the cartilaginous phases of bone repair that correlates with a decrease in IHH signaling. The authors concluded mechanical stabilization influences mesenchymal cell differentiation to bone.[11] Because the mechanical stabilization is under the control of surgeons and it can affect signaling pathways important for bone healing, this aspect of fracture stabilization is key in minimizing nonunions.

AUTOGRAFT

Autograft often comes to mind as being the gold standard for bone grafting because of its osteogenic and osteoconductive properties. Autograft does not contain a significant amount of bone morphogenetic protein (BMP), so it is not considered osteoinductive.[3] The most common site for autograft is the iliac crest. Other sites to consider are the greater trochanter, proximal tibia at Gerdy's tubercle, distal tibia, the distal radius, and olecranon.[9] Autograft contains rich sources of progenitor cells and growth factors, which are essential to help in the healing process. With cancellous bone grafts, about 15% of the osteoblasts and osteocytes survive and are capable of producing early bone.[3,12] The surface area of the cancellous bone allows ingrowth of blood vessels and influx of osteoblast precursors. There is an active process of bone formation and resorption with eventual remodeling of the new bone.

After the autogenous cancellous cell bone is placed at the nonunion site and there is bleeding bone induced by taking down the nonunion, the cascade to promote healing begins. There are vascular buds that infiltrate the site and the graft is surrounded by inflammatory cells.[9] If nonsteroidal anti-inflammatories are used during this phase, they would reduce the inflammatory response and thus inhibit the bone-forming cells. A small amount of fibrous tissue is formed later in the second week.[9] In the fibrous granulation tissue predominant at the recipient nonunion site, there is an increase in osteoclastic activity observed.[9] The macrophages remove necrotic tissue within the Haversian canals of the graft and there are intracellular by-products, which attract undifferentiated stem cells.[4]

The secondary phase of cancellous incorporation involves osteoblasts lining the edges of the trabeculi and laying down a seam of osteoid, which surrounds the necrotic bone.[9] The necrotic bone is gradually resorbed by osteoclasts.[3] New bone continues to form. Then bone remodeling occurs over several months in response to the stresses placed on the bone.

Autograft can be an ideal choice in an aseptic nonunion in a healthy, young patient. You know the source of graft, and if there are no concerns regarding bone quality or metabolic deficiencies, autograft is a viable choice. The fracture has mechanical stability and needs a good biologic environment. By taking down the nonunion to a healthy tissue bed, autograft can provide the osteoconductive and osteogenic properties to promote healing.

With autograft, there are complications to consider in up to 40% of patients.[3,9,12] These complications include limited donor site availability and donor site morbidities, which may include pain, iatrogenic fracture, and the need for increased hospital stay (which affects the economics of fracture care). With advancing technology and choices available for bone graft substitute, autograft may no longer be the gold standard.

BONE MARROW ASPIRATE

Because we know the success of autograft, the consideration for obtaining cells from the iliac crest through a bone marrow aspirate became highly attractive in terms of minimizing complications involved in the harvesting of the bone graft. This is not a new concept. In 1869, Goujon demonstrated the osteogenic capacity of bone marrow.[4,13] The potency of the osteogenic capabilities of the bone marrow was considered.[14] It is known the quality of this is donor dependent. The marrow has been estimated to contain 1/50,000 nucleated stem cells in younger adults and 1/1,000,000 in the elderly.[4] Thus, women older than 35 with osteoporotic bone and/or elderly patients can have fewer stem cells available for formation of bone.[13] In addition, with the increased knowledge of nonunions having a metabolic deficiency, we would be harvesting bone marrow from someone who is metabolically deficient.[5]

If this material is injected, concerns include localization of the aspirate in the desired area. In addition, the studies published describe injecting the bone marrow aspirate directly into the nonunion without taking down the nonunion and preparing a bed to accept a bone graft substitute.[13–15] Connolly and colleagues[15] reported on the use of autologous bone marrow injection in 20 ununited tibial fractures over a 5-year period. This technique was used in conjunction with either a cast or an intramedullary (IM) nail fixation. The authors felt that the marrow stimulated callous formation significant enough to unite 8 of 10 nonunions mobilized with cast and 10 of 10 fractures treated with IM nails. Thus the authors concluded that the bone marrow injection was just as effective as autogenous bone grafting.[15] There were confounding variables in this study. Because there was some mechanical stability provided at the same time, it makes it difficult to know which intervention, the aspirate or treatment chosen, was responsible for the results. In addition, in closely evaluating the results, the percutaneous bone marrow injection did not promote bone healing any more rapidly than with standard grafting, as it took an average time to healing of 6 months after injection.[15]

Once the marrow is obtained, it needs to be processed to maximize its osteoinductivity. Different centrifugation techniques may affect the amounts of bone formation. Hernigou and colleagues[13] evaluated percutaneous autologous bone marrow grafting for tibial nonunions specifically regarding the number of cells, number in concentration of progenitor cells transplanted, and callous volume and healing. They aspirated the bone marrow for 60 noninfected atrophic nonunions. The bone marrow was directly injected into the site without taking down any fibrous tissue and the overall results found that the aspirate contained an average of 612 ± 134 progenitor cells before concentration and an average of 2579 ± 1120 progenitors per cubic cm after concentration.[13] In addition, the authors evaluated the fibroblast colony forming units (CFU) injected into each nonunion. There was bone union achieved in 53 patients and the bone marrow that was injected into the nonunion of the patient group that healed contained greater than 1500 progenitors per cubic cm.[13] They found that the concentration and number injected into the nonunion sites of the patients without healing was significantly lower. The authors acknowledge the variability in osteogenic potential from patient to patient. Thus, the amount of progenitor cells is related to the effectiveness of percutaneous autologous bone marrow grafting. The authors cannot explain a mechanism to account for transformation of fibrous tissue into callous; normally the other fibrous nonunion needs to be taken out. It is like putting a band-aid on a laceration requiring sutures and getting lucky when it heals.

Watson and colleagues[16] evaluated iliac crest aspirate of delayed union and nonunion of long bones in 52 patients over an 8-year period. The patients were aspirated under general anesthesia and the aspirate was centrifuged, the cellular concentrate was obtained, and large-bore needles were directed at the site of bone deficit under fluoroscopy. There were 46 patients available for long-term follow-up over 2 years. The results were quite poor with only 17 (37%) achieving bony union after the first procedure with an average time to union of 4 months after intervention. Two patients healed their nonunion after a second procedure and 6 of 7 patients who received multiple injections had a persistent nonunion despite these procedures. Of a total of 56 procedures performed, 37 (66%) failed.[16] There was no difference between the group that healed versus the group that did not heal with regard to gender, fracture treatment, smoking, or type of nonunion. The use of iliac crest aspiration injection alone was found to be ineffective in the treatment of nonunion.

The studies discussed provide variable results. The effectiveness of the bone marrow aspirate is dependent on the donor, and if the donor already demonstrated an inability to heal, one must wonder about the benefits of this procedure. The use of percutaneous bone marrow aspirate as a bone graft substitute at this time is not promising or supported by high level of evidence studies.

PLATELET CONCENTRATE

As we discussed, fracture repair involves a process in which you get formation of a blood clot and an environment rich in growth factors to promote healing. So thus the natural thought is that with fracture, the platelets activated and granules released contain many osteopromotive factors.[4,5] So the thought extended to using platelet-derived growth factor (PDGF) and platelet-rich plasma (PRP) to help promote healing. It was thought if one could deliver the platelets in a concentrated amount this would theoretically contribute to earlier bone repair and fracture healing. Platelets are isolated from autologous blood and this eliminates the concern for any immune response. The PRP therapy has been used since the 1970s.[17] So the question became if this therapy is used by itself or in addition to bone graft material, could this promote healing?

PDGF/PRP are osteopromotive products, not osteoinductive products, and the concentration of the growth factors varies.[5] Proteases used in the preparation of the product may degrade the growth factors.[17] The machines used can destroy the platelets. In addition, PRP is often used in combination with allograft and/or autograft composites. Recent studies found that although components of PRP stimulate migration and proliferation of osteogenic progenitor cells, they also inhibit the osteogenic action of BMPs.[17,18]

Because PDGF and PRP are often used in conjunction with other products in bone grafting, they were evaluated combined with demineralized bone matrix (DBM) in immunocompromised mice. The authors found that PDGF inhibited bone formation in a dose-dependent manner.[18] PRP also reduced the osteoinductivity of the DBM.[18]

The role of PRP in osteoinductive promotion of bone healing is not promising at this time. The product may have osteopromotive factors and has been found to be effective in certain types of surgery; specifically in wound healing and also in oral maxillofacial surgery. We continue to emphasize the importance of the surrounding tissue in healing of nonunions. The environment in oral maxillofacial surgery is different. The bone is different and subjected to different stresses, and it may be that PRP/PDGF may be enough to promote bone healing. However, the environment in which bone healing is required in humans after fracture repair is different. Most often it is in the diaphysial region and not like the rich cancellous bone in the oral maxillofacial region. In addition, PDGF/PRP may be helpful in wound healing, whether or not this effect helps with fracture healing is not proven at this time.

VASCULAR ENDOTHELIAL GROWTH FACTOR

In evaluating which factors are present after an injury that may promote healing, VEGF has shown some potential; however, there needs to be significantly more research in this area. The premise is that with fractures there is a hematoma that forms, and there are signaling peptides and angiogenic growth factors that are released. We know a good angiogenic environment can promote healing and is necessary for survival of the bone graft. One of the most potent angiogenic growth factors is VEGF,[19,20] which stimulates the formation of the new blood vessels. However, VEGF does not appear to be directly involved in osteoblast differentiation. So, thus, the bone-forming cells are recruited through another mechanism, perhaps the pericyte circulating cytokines, the blood clot, and the fractured bone ends.[20]

Eckardt and colleagues[20] studied rabbit nonunions and VEGF was found to enhance bone healing. All rabbit nonunions treated with VEGF and autograft healed. VEGF stimulated the formation of competent bone in an environment that did not have the ability to heal, as it was stripped of its vascularization and of its blood supply. Although VEGF appears to provide some promise in coupling angiogenesis in a healthy environment to bone healing, the applicability of this still remains to be seen as there must be significant evidence presented. The use of VEGF emphasizes the importance of the environment to promote bone healing.

DEMINERALIZED BONE MATRIX

DBM is often advertised by the multiple manufacturers that produce it as osteoinductive. It is important to understand the research behind it and its role in bone healing. DBM is prepared from cadaveric human bone and it is available from multiple vendors in multiple preparations including gel, putties, or strips. DBM is an acid extraction of the cadaveric human bone leaving the noncollagenous proteins, which include bone morphogenetic proteins, bone growth factors, and type 1 collagen.[3-5] The processing may decrease the availability of the bone morphogenetic protein and quality of product.[3-5] In addition, it is important to consider that there is significant donor variability in the DBM.

DBM is often used in combination with cancellous bone and other substitutes. It is used in metaphyseal bone to fill bone defects and cysts; as an autologous bone graft expander as a composite graft with bone marrow and other substitutes. However, the research reporting its use in nonunions and in spinal fusion does not support a high level of osteoinductivity. The human data are inconclusive. There are many isolated case reports and Level 4 evidence studies.

DBM is acellular and its success depends on the cellular environment of the host bone. The Food and Drug Administration (FDA) allowed DBM to be produced without significant regulation. Currently the DBMs are in a pathway that does not require demonstration of efficacy compared with autografts. Now the FDA plans to regulate DBM as a class II medical device, which has more stringent regulations in terms of product and its efficacy.[3]

It is important to understand the limitations of DBM. It has very mild osteoinductivity. Less than 5% of DBM is composed of growth factors. Blum and colleagues[21] showed bone formation depends on the amount of the RhBMP-2 in the demineralized bone matrix. They tested 113 lots of demineralized bone matrix and found that RhBMP-2 quantities varied from 200 to 6744 picograms per gram.[21] Thus, there is significant variability in the lots of the DBM testing.

In addition, in a spine fusion model in athymic rats, three different brands of demineralized bone matrix were tested. There was one group that had higher radiographic fusion and histologically the most new bone formation. So this study demonstrated there is a difference in osteoinductive potentials for the DBM products available in the animal model.[22]

We know about the inherent variability of the donor, we know that there are differences in the commercial products, and there are low level evidence studies supporting its use in fracture repair. The questions are what is the role of DBM in promoting healing and what are the factors that it possesses to promote healing? DBM contains the bone morphogenetic proteins, and the amount of new bone that will be formed is directly related to the amount of bone morphogenetic protein present in the product; however, that is not something we know ahead of time.

DBM was shown to be just as effective as autograft in a humeral nonunion model.[23] In this case series, DBM was just as effective as autograft; however, it was placed in an excellent environment with the soft tissue surrounding and in a fracture that has a high rate of healing with the treatment (plating) of nonunions.

In summary, if DBM is used, realize that it has limited osteoinductivity and most often it is used with other bone graft substitutes; however, there is nothing proven with high-level evidence in fracture nonunions or spinal fusions. No good prospective studies prove the benefits of DBM, but perhaps with the combination of products it is used with it would not hinder the survival of bone graft substitutes.

BONE MORPHOGENETIC PROTEINS

The osteoinductivity of bone morphogenetic proteins has exciting implications in fracture and nonunion care. BMPs have been used and studied extensively for the past several years. Marshall Urist in 1965 discovered that DBM induces new bone formation. By 1971, he coined the term bone morphogenetic protein. In 1977, he discovered that BMP extracted from bone is osteoinductive.[5] It took several years and lots of science and technology but in 1988, the first recombinant human bone morphogenetic protein was produced. This was very promising because it allowed for increased production of the BMP and studying of the product. Marshall Urist stated that "Bone morphogenetic protein allows osteogenesis to be under the control of surgeons."[24]

The whole process of how BMPs work has been analyzed extensively. Preclinical studies have characterized a cascade of cellular events involved in the bone-forming process. In the first step, BMP attracts cells to the site of implantation. In vitro studies have demonstrated that BMP causes a chemotactic migration of bone-forming cells to the site of local concentration.[25] The exposure to BMPs causes cell-specific proliferation of undifferentiated human mesenchymal stem cells.[26,27] A BMP bonds the specific receptors on the stem cell surface causing them to differentiate into the bone-forming osteoblast.[28] There are more than 14 bone morphogenetic proteins characterized but not all BMPs are capable of this binding. Cheng and colleagues[29] analyzed the osteogenetic activity of 14 types of BMPs. BMPs 2, 6, and 9 were found to play an important role in inducing osteoblastic differentiation of mesenchymal stem cells. BMPs 2, 6, and 9 are active on the stem cells to the preosteoblast, and then BMPs 2, 4, 7, and 9

are quite active from the preosteoblast to the osteoblast stage.[29]

The osteoblasts form new bone and the body remodels this new bone in response to the environmental and mechanical forces. It is important to realize when implanting BMPs, it is not a magic potion. There needs to be an acceptable biologic and mechanical environment for healing.

There are two commercially available recombinant BMPs available for use. The first one discussed is RhBMP-7, marketed as OP1 by Stryker Biotech. The RhBMP-7 has received a humanitarian device exception (HDE) from the FDA for nonunion in tibia fractures. With an HDE, the device is not required to demonstrate superior effectiveness to autograft. The manufacturer must demonstrate safety. The surgeon must get institutional review board approval before using the product and it could be used only in emergency off label and the manufacturer must be notified. The FDA limits the use of its product on an annual basis. This HDE is based on the results of a prospective randomized trial of 122 patients with 124 tibial nonunion with 9 months of follow-up.[30] There had been prior reaming and nailing in 43% of the RhBMP-7 patients and 31% of the allograft patients. There was radiographic healing in 75% of the OP1 patients, and 84% of the allograft patients.[30] At 9 months, 81% of the RhBMP-7 patients and 85% of the allograft patients were determined to have clinical success. RhBMP-7 also has a spine HDE.

A recent article evaluated RhBMP-7 in distal tibial fractures treated with an external fixator.[31] There were 20 patients with a control group treated with the hybrid external fixator. They found more fractures healed at 16 to 20 weeks with RhBMP-7. Also, the time to union, time off work, and duration of the external fixator in place was less with the RhBMP-7 group.[30] Two patients from the RhBMP-7 group and seven in the control group required secondary interventions.

McKee and colleagues[32] evaluated the effectiveness of RhBMP-7 on the healing of open tibial shaft fractures over 124 patients at seven university centers. There were 62 controls and 62 received RhBMP-7. All patients were appropriate for IM nailing and randomized to standard wound closure or closure with the addition of RhBMP-7. All patients received irrigation and debridement of the open fractures and historically locked nail. The results demonstrated no RhBMP-7 adverse events. Seventeen patients in the control group and eight in the RhBMP-7 group needed a secondary intervention ($P = .02$).[32] The authors found improved functional outcome in the RhBMP-7 group with 80% reporting good outcome compared with 56% in the allograft group.

RhBMP-2 is marketed as Infuse by Medtronic Sofamer Danek in Memphis, Tennessee. Its carrier is an absorbable collagen sponge (ACS), which binds the bone morphogenetic protein for local delivery.[33] This is in contrast to RhBMP-7, which is injected into the area used with no carrier sponge. RhBMP-2 has received FDA approval in spine for anterior interbody fusions with a specific implant, and also for oral and maxillofacial surgery use as a bone graft substitute in alveolar ridge reconstruction. In addition, RhBM-2 has an FDA-approved indication in trauma for open tibia fractures. The FDA approved RhBMP-2 in 2004 for use in open tibial fractures with intramedullary nail and implantation of the RhBMP-2 within 14 days. The full prospective randomized clinical study of 450 patients with open tibia fractures was reported in 2002. There were three groups: a control group receiving IM nail and no RhBMP-2 (Standard of Care [SOC]), a lower dose of RhBMP-2 at 0.75 mg/mL, and a higher dose of RhBMP@ at 1.5 mg/mL. The low dose group did better than the control (SOC) but not as well as the higher dose group. Only results from the control patients and the investigational patients receiving the dosing of RhBMP-2 at 1.5 mg/mL are described as part of the FDA effectiveness evaluation.

The BMP-2 Evaluation in Surgery for Tibial Trauma (BESTT) study group was a prospective randomized control study, with randomization of 150 control patients with open tibia fractures to treatment with intramedullary nail (SOC) and wound closure and 149 with the standard of care and RhBM-2.[34] The patients were followed for 12 months after definitive wound closure and assessment was made by clinical and radiographic review. The primary end point was bone healing. Failure was defined as those patients who required a secondary intervention to promote healing. The secondary intervention rate was significantly lower in the RhBMP-2 bone graft group as compared with the standard of care group. The reduction in secondary intervention was 41%, as 44% of the SOC and 26% of the RhBMP-2 group required secondary intervention.[34] The rate of nonunion was lower in the RhBMP-2 group as compared with the controls. Union was defined as no secondary intervention and radiographic healing of the fracture. There were a total of 80 in the control group and 56 in the RhBMP-2 group who were considered nonunion. This represented a 29% reduction in the risk of nonunion ($P<.0075$).[34] Although it is important to realize the overall nonunion rate of 53% is high, this was based on the strict definitions as necessitated by governing bodies for approval of this drug. Another beneficial outcome found in this study was that the combined rate of deep and superficial infections was lower in patients with Gustilo 3A and 3B fractures in the RhBMP-2 group as compared with the control group. A 44% reduction in infection risk was noted ($P = .0377$).[34] It should be noted that the RhBMP-2 does not directly prevent infection from occurring; however, because of the angiogenic response with the use of RhBMP-2, the rate of infection may be decreased by having an adequate blood supply in the area.

RhBMP-2 was evaluated in tibial fractures with bone loss in a prospective randomized study comparing open or closed fractures that required a staged reconstruction.[35] There were 30 patients total in the study: 15 received RhBMP-2 and allograft and 15 received autogenous bone graft. Two patients in the RhBMP-2 group required a secondary intervention and four in the autogenous bone graft group required a secondary intervention including one patient who was not healed at 12 months. Secondary intervention was considered a treatment failure as in the previous study. Overall, it was concluded that there was comparable rate of healing, fewer donor site complaints with the use of RhBMP-2, and less blood loss in the RhBMP-2 group.[35] Thus, the authors concluded that RhBMP-2 is a reasonable alternative to autogenous bone graft. However, this is not considered on-label use of the device by the FDA.

Bone morphogenetic proteins represent an exciting option in the treatment of fractures because of their potent osteoinductivity. They are not a magic potion. The use of these products as a bone graft substitute requires the appropriate biology and mechanical stability. The future is promising as we see Marshall Urist's wishes of bringing bone healing under the control of surgeons come to reality.

SUMMARY

The healing of fractures and nonunions has significant science background to it; however, the application of the products in the surgeon's hands should be considered an art in the science of bone healing. The surgeon must choose the adequate fixation for stability and to promote healing by not making the construct too stiff. The surgeon must choose the type of bone graft substitute depending on patient factors and surgeon factors involving the treatment of the fracture.

REFERENCES

1. Tsiridis E, Upadhyay N, Giannoudis P. Molecular aspects of fracture healing: which are the important molecules? Injury 2007;38(Suppl 1):S11–25.
2. Bielby R, Jones E, McGonagle D. The role of mesenchymal stem cells in maintenance and repair of bone. Injury 2007;38(Suppl 1):S26–32.
3. Brown CR, Boden SD. Fracture repair and bone grafting. In: Fischgrund JS, editor. Orthopaedic knowledge update 9. Rosemont (IL): AAOS; 2008. p. 13–22.
4. Khan SN, Cammisa FP Jr, Sandhu HS, et al. The biology of bone grafting. J Am Acad Orthop Surg 2005;13(1):77–86.
5. De Long WG Jr, Einhorn TA, Koval K, et al. Bone grafts and bone graft substitutes in orthopaedic trauma surgery. A critical analysis. J Bone Joint Surg Am 2007;89(3):649–58.
6. Cannada LK, Anglen JO, Archdeacon MT, et al. Avoiding complications in the care of fractures of the tibia. J Bone Joint Surg Am 2008;90(8): 1760–8.
7. Brinker MR, O'Connor DP, Monla YT, et al. Metabolic and endocrine abnormalities in patients with nonunions. J Orthop Trauma 2007;21(8):557–70.
8. Gaston P, Will E, Elton RA, et al. Fractures of the tibia. Can their outcome be predicted? J Bone Joint Surg Br 1999;81(1):71–6.
9. Sen MK, Miclau T. Autologous iliac crest bone graft: should it still be the gold standard for treating nonunions? Injury 2007;38(Suppl 1):S75–80.
10. Jahangir AA, Nunley RM, Mehta S, et al. Bone graft substitutes in orthopaedic surgery. J Am Acad Orthop Surg Now 2008;2(1):35–7.
11. Le AX, Miclau T, Hu D, et al. Molecular aspects of healing in stabilized and non-stabilized fractures. J Orthop Res 2001;19(1):78–84.
12. Ebraheim NA, Elgafy H, Xu R. Bone-graft harvesting from iliac and fibular donor sites: techniques and complications. J Am Acad Orthop Surg 2001;9(3): 210–8.
13. Hernigou P, Poignard A, Beaujean F, et al. Percutaneous autologous bone-marrow grafting for nonunions. Influence of the number and concentration of progenitor cells. J Bone Joint Surg Am 2005;87(7):1430–7.
14. Burwell RG. The function of bone marrow in the incorporation of a bone graft. Clin Orthop Relat Res 1985;200:125–41.
15. Connolly JF, Guse R, Tiedeman J, et al. Autologous marrow injection as a substitute for operative grafting of tibial nonunions. Clin Orthop Relat Res 1991; 266:259–70.
16. Watson JT, Quigley KJ, Mudd CD. Percutaneous injection of iliac crest aspirate for the treatment of long bone delayed union and nonunion. Orthopaedic Trauma Association annual meeting, Phoenix (AZ), Paper #13, Oct 5–7, 2006.
17. Boyan BD, Schwartz Z, Patterson TE, et al. Clinical use of platelet rich plasma on orthopaedics. J Am Acad Orthop Surg Now 2007;1(9):44–6.
18. Ranly DM, McMillan J, Keller T, et al. Platelet derived growth factor inhibits demineralized bone matrix induced intramuscular cartilage and bone formation. J Bone Joint Surg Am 2005;87(9): 2052–64.
19. Deckers MM, van Bezooijen RL, van der Horst G, et al. Bone morphogenetic proteins stimulate angiogenesis through osteoblast-derived vascular endothelial growth factor A. Endocrinology 2002;143(4): 1545–53.
20. Eckardt H, Ding M, Hansen ES, et al. Recombinant human vascular endothelial growth factor enhances bone healing in an experimental model. J Bone Joint Surg Br 2005;87(10):1434–8.
21. Blum B, Moseley J, Miller L, et al. Measurement of bone morphogenetic proteins and other growth factors in demineralized bone matrix. Orthopedics 2004;27(1 Suppl):s161–5.
22. Peterson B, Whang PG, Iglesias R, et al. Osteoinductivity of commercially available demineralized bone matrix. Preparations in a spine fusion model. J Bone Joint Surg Am 2004;86(10): 2243–50.
23. Hierholzer C, Sama D, Toro JB, et al. Plate fixation of ununited humeral shaft fractures: effect of type of bone graft on healing. J Bone Joint Surg Am 2006; 88(7):1442–7.
24. Urist MR. Bone morphogenetic protein: the molecularization of skeletal system development. J Bone Miner Res 1997;12(3):343–6.
25. Fiedler J, Röderer G, Günther KP, et al. BMP-2, BMP-4, and PDGF-bb stimulate chemotactic migration of primary human mesenchymal progenitor cells. J Cell Biochem 2002;87(3): 305–12.
26. Akita S, Fukui M, Nakagawa H, et al. Cranial bone defect healing is accelerated by mesenchymal stem cells induced by coadministration of bone morphogenetic protein-2 and basic fibroblast growth factor. Wound Repair Regen 2004;12(2): 252–9.
27. Wilke A, Traub F, Kienapfel H, et al. Cell differentiation under the influence of RhBMP-2. Biochem Biophys Res Commun 2001;284(5):1093–7.
28. Akino K, Mineta T, Fukui M, et al. Bone morphogenetic protein-2 regulates proliferation of human mesenchymal stem cells. Wound Repair Regen 2003;11(5):354–60.
29. Cheng H, Jiang W, Phillips FM, et al. Osteogenic activity of the fourteen types of human bone morphogenetic proteins (BMPs). J Bone Joint Surg Am 2003;85(8):1544–52.

30. Friedlaender GE, Perry CR, Cole JD, et al. Osteo-genic protein-1 (bone morphogenetic protein-7) in the treatment of tibial nonunions. J Bone Joint Surg Am 2001;83(Suppl 1(Pt 2)):S151–8.

31. Ristiniemi J, Flinkkilä T, Hyvönen P, et al. RhBMP-7 accelerates the healing in distal tibial fractures treated by external fixation. J Bone Joint Surg Br 2007;89(2):265–72.

32. McKee MD, Schemitsch EH, Waddell JP, et al. The effect of human recombinant bone morphogenic protein (RhBMP-7) on the healing of open tibial shaft fractures: results of a multi-center, prospective, randomized clinical trial. Presented at the 2002 OTA Annual Meeting, Toronto (Canada), October 12, 2002.

33. Riedel GE, Valentin-Opran A. Clinical evaluation of RhBMP-2/ACS in orthopedic trauma: a progress report. Orthopedics 1999;22(7):663–5.

34. Govender S, Csimma C, Genant HK, et al. Recombinant human bone morphogenetic protein-2 for treatment of open tibial fractures: a prospective, controlled, randomized study of four hundred and fifty patients. J Bone Joint Surg Am 2002;84(12):2123–34.

35. Jones AL, Bucholz RW, Bosse MJ, et al. Recombinant human BMP-2 and allograft compared with autogenous bone graft for reconstruction of diaphyseal tibial fractures with cortical defects. A randomized, controlled trial. J Bone Joint Surg Am 2006;88(7):1431–41.

Use of Solid and Cancellous Autologous Bone Graft for Fractures and Nonunions

James T. Marino, MD, Bruce H. Ziran, MD*

KEYWORDS
- Autograft • Bone loss • Nonunion • Autologous • Iliac crest

Bone is the second most commonly implanted material in the human body, after blood transfusion, with an estimated 600,000 grafts performed annually. Although the market for bone graft substitutes is more than $1 billion, that of bone graft itself is still more than half that amount.[1,2] Reports of autologous bone grafting date back to the ancient Egyptians, yet the modern scientific study of grafting began in the early 19th century. Since then, the indications, methodology, and science of bone grafts in nonunion and bone loss have been established and refined, and new methods of harvesting and treatment are being developed and implemented. This article describes the use of solid and cancellous bone graft in the treatment of acute bone loss and nonunion.

The modern study of bone grafting can traced back to the work of Ollier[3] in the mid-1800s, when he showed that transplanted bone could be osteogenic (although some earlier work examined the osteogenic qualities of bone). Nearly 50 years later in 1914, Phemister[4] showed what occurs to a graft when transplanted. He found that some of the transplanted cells survive at the endosteal or periosteal surface, but that the deeper cells die. Also, over time older bone is replaced by newly formed bone. This process, the remodeling by osteoclastic resorption and creation of new vascular channels with osteoblastic bone formation, would progress to become what is now defined as *creeping substitution*.

In other clinical studies, Phemister described a novel technique with excellent results of onlay bone grafting, in which a pocket is created around the recipient site through lifting an osteoperiosteal sleeve with slivers of cortical bone. The graft is placed within this created space and the ununited fracture callus is left undisturbed, the latter concept going against the prevailing practice at the time (**Fig. 1**).[5]

Judet and Judet[6] described another method for exposing onlay bone graft to vascularize host tissue, wherein the cortical surface of the bone was elevated with an osteotome in what is best described as *fish scaling*. In this method, the outer cortex is lifted to expose the graft to underlying haversian canals and cortical capillary bleeding (**Fig. 2**).

Further advancing the technique of bone grafting, in 1945 Harmon[7] described the technique still commonly used today of posterolateral grafting for nonunion of the tibia. The goal was to create a synostosis between the tibia and the fibula. This method provided considerable advantage over previous methods. Through placing the graft posterior, potentially compromised soft tissue or infection is avoided anteriorly, and the improved vascular supply of the posterior musculature leads to faster graft incorporation (**Fig. 3**).

The understanding of bone graft physiology advanced significantly with Urist's[8] work in 1965 when he showed the capacity of devitalized bone matrix to induce bone formation in heterotopic sites. In further experimentation, Urist[8] and colleagues[9] identified *bone morphogenic protein* (BMP), a substance they believed was capable of

Department of Orthopedic Surgery, Atlanta Medical Center, 303 Parkway Drive NE, Atlanta, GA 30312, USA
* Corresponding author.
E-mail address: bruce.ziran@tenethealth.com (B.H. Ziran).

Orthop Clin N Am 41 (2010) 15–26
doi:10.1016/j.ocl.2009.08.003
0030-5898/09/$ – see front matter © 2010 Elsevier Inc. All rights reserved.

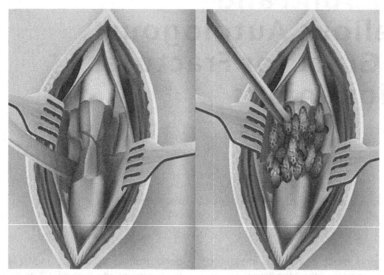

Fig. 1. Judet method of osteoperiosteal elevation to create a pocket to place local bone graft.

signaling the differentiation of mesenchymal cells into cartilage and bone. Studies have now shown more than 40 different BMPs. The commercially available BMP products (BMP2 and BMP7) are in wide clinical use and discussed elsewhere in this issue.

Today, experts understand that Urist's early work identified the processes of osteoinductivity, osteoconductivity, and osteogenicity. Osteoinduction is the process through which a signal is sent to influence the formation of new bone. The aptly named BMPs have been shown to play a significant role in this process, but many other molecules and proteins (eg, transforming growth factor beta) are involved in the process. Osteoconduction refers to the scaffolding over which new bone must grow for healing to occur. The properties of the scaffold, such as material, pore size, and porosity, can influence the rate of incorporation of a bone graft. Osteogenesis is the graft's ability to form bone by way of its cellular elements, whether through differentiation of mesenchymal cells or recruitment of osteoblasts and osteocytes. Autologous bone graft remains the gold standard because it is believed to contain all three characteristics.

Fundamental to the discussion of bone graft is an overview of bone formation, fracture healing, and graft incorporation. Bone is formed in one of two ways. Endochondral ossification involves the creation of a cartilage model of bone that is secondarily used by osteoblasts as a template for bone formation. The steps are chondrocyte proliferation, chondrocyte hypertrophy, matrix mineralization, apoptosis, vascular invasion, ossification, and remodeling to lamellar bone. This process is how long bones are formed.

Intramembranous ossification avoids the use of a calcified cartilage template and relies on the direct formation of bone matrix by osteoblasts. This process is responsible for the formation of flat bones and for the growth in width of the long bones.

Fracture healing involves both types of bone formation to varying degrees, depending on stability at the fracture site. High stability results in direct osteonal healing (also known as *direct* or *primary*) bone formation, which is similar to intramembranous healing. In the setting of lower stability (motion at the fracture site), endochondral (also known as *indirect* or *secondary*) bone formation occurs. In vivo, fracture healing typically involves a combination of these processes.[9,10]

A major consideration in healing and bone grafting is the viability and vascularity of the tissue bed, because the recipient site plays a major role in

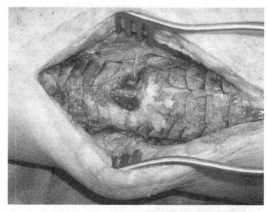

Fig. 2. Phemister method of scaling the cortex to expose the onlay graft to the microvasculature of the bone.

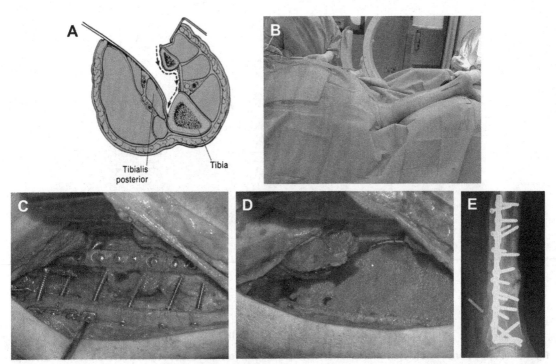

Fig. 3. (*A*) Anatomic planes used for posterolateral bone grafting. The interval follows the posterior fibula across the interosseous membrane to the tibia. This exposure becomes more difficult in the proximal aspects of the tibia. (*B*) Illustration showing the position of the patient for posterolateral bone grafting, along with the preparation to harvest autograft from the posterior iliac crest. (*C*) Intraoperative image of the exposure along with adjunct fixation. In some cases, the fibula was used as a laterally based strut to help support the tibia. Because of the fixed angles of the bicortical screws in the fibula, they functioned similarly to the current locked plating technology. (*D*) Intraoperative image of the graft material covering and spanning both tibia and fibula. (*E*) Radiograph of a posterolateral graft at 8 months after it has healed and incorporated. Note that anterior defects may be well tolerated if an adequate posterior consolidation is achieved.

determining the success of grafting. The results of bone healing and grafting in various anatomic sites reflect this concept. The femur and forearm uncommonly have healing problems because they have a well-vascularized muscle envelope. The distal tibia, however, remains the nemesis of the fracture surgeon.

Aside from the limb segment, the anatomic site within a given bone, whether diaphyseal or metaphyseal, will also influence the needs of a graft. A contained metaphyseal defect is vascular and surrounded by host bone, with a greater surface area to which a graft can consolidate. The contained defect, through exposure to local host bone, will also have access to local bone cells, making recruitment of osteogenic cells easier.

A diaphyseal defect is usually uncontained and may not even have a healthy muscle envelope at its margins. Therefore, any graft placed into such a hostile environment will first require a potent angiogenic influence, followed by a chemotactic element to recruit appropriate osteogenic cells before bone formation. The authors' decision algorithm for bone graft use centers on the viability of the tissue bed, nature of the defect, and structural needs.

A contained metaphyseal defect does not generally need potent graft material such as autograft, and can be well treated with alternative methods such as allograft or synthetic cements. Conversely, in segmental bone loss, which has poor vascularity and osteogenic potential, an autogenous bone graft remains the gold standard.

Nonunions can be subdivided into hypertrophic, oligotrophic, and atrophic types, which guides the needed intervention to achieve healing. Hypertrophic and oligotrophic nonunions are similar in that they have biologic potential, with a blood supply sufficient to allow for healing (**Fig. 4**). Although the former is usually caused by a lack of fracture stability and is characterized by large amounts of callus formation, the latter exhibits little callous at the fracture site, often because of poor fracture reduction or inadequate bone contact.

Hypertrophic nonunions require stability, and when this is provided, they achieve bony union quickly, without the need for any bone grafting or

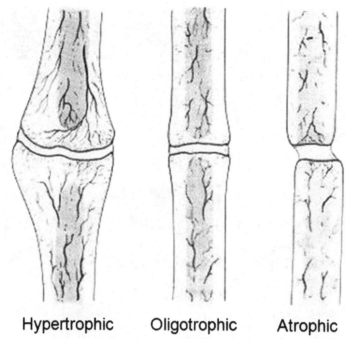

Hypertrophic   Oligotrophic   Atrophic

Fig. 4. The appearance of different nonunions. Attempted bone formation about the fracture site is an attempt to stabilize the site and shows biologic capacity. Lack of any bone formation suggests the lack of vascularity and biologic potential.

biologic augmentation. Oligotrophic nonunion treatment frequently involves improving fragment alignment, with bone grafting performed selectively, depending on the condition of the bone bed and surrounding soft tissue envelope. If the bone and soft tissue envelope are disrupted during the process of achieving appropriate alignment and stabilization, then bone grafting should be considered because an iatrogenic lowering of the biologic potential has occurred. If the alignment and stabilization can be achieved biologically, then bone grafting could be optional and depends on the judgment of the surgeon.

Atrophic nonunions are an entirely different entity. They lack a sufficient blood supply and are located within a zone of injury that frequently has other damaged structures. The atrophic nonunion is lacking biologic potential and requires bone grafting, with the autograft still the gold standard. In cases that also require structural support, cortical autograft can be used, but in many of these situations, surgeons may choose to use a structural allograft or synthetic core with a surrounding biologic autograft to encourage a bridging osseous connection. In the atrophic nonunion and potentially in the oligotrophic nonunion, the decortication methods described previously are needed to stimulate a new healing response from the local host bone and expose the graft bone to a bleeding osseous surface.[11]

The discussion of autologous grafting for acute bone loss and nonunion would not be complete without the mention of distraction osteogenesis. Distraction osteogenesis was pioneered by the Russian Gavril Ilizarov[12] in the 1960s. He found that bone can form new bone when it is gently distracted by up to 1 mm/d. Large bone defects have been successfully treated with this method. In general, the phenomenon of distraction osteogenesis is most similar to intramembranous ossification, and although some unique differences have been noted, their discussion is not within the scope of this article. Unfortunately, the tissue that forms between distracted bone ends is soft and requires a period of secondary support to allow the regenerated bone to mature. This method of autograft, although having distinct disadvantages and morbidity for other reasons, does not have much donor site morbidity, is an excellent form of autograft, and may actually be the ultimate autograft.

Another method of autologous grafting involves the use of bone marrow aspirates. Although technically not bone, the graft is generally obtained from the pelvis to obtain the same autologous inductive proteins and osteogenic cells found in pelvic autografts. Both osteogenic and osteoinductive cells and factors are present in the marrow aspirate. Therefore, theoretically, if they are combined with allograft or similar bone graft substitute, the resulting combination should be similar to autogenous cancellous graft.

This theoretical claim has not been shown in scientific clinical studies. One possible reason is that autogenous bone itself may harbor certain elements that allogenic bone does not (lost during its procurement and processing). Additionally, bone marrow aspirate contains a variable number of osteoprogenitor cells depending on several factures, including age, sex, and harvesting technique.

Studies that have promoted bone marrow aspirate for nonunions described their use in stable nonunions, implying that the nonunions were hypertrophic or oligotrophic.[13,14] By virtue of being a stable nonunion, they may potentially have healed without the use of bone marrow aspirate and therefore may not be extrapolated for use in an atrophic nonunion. Furthermore, most nonunion sites do not contain readily created spaces around the bone and are usually surrounded by dense fibrous tissue. They require the creation of a potential space around the site, and would also benefit from some type of surface preparation of the site to facilitate an interaction between the marrow elements and local host tissue. The authors have not found bone marrow aspirate alone to be useful, but believe it may be a complementary ingredient when combined with other factors during an open procedure.

The technique of harvesting bone marrow aspirate is important to optimize osteogenic element, otherwise most of the aspirate may contain only hematopoietic elements that would not be useful for bone healing. A recent study showed an average of 1 in 20,000 cells, with a range of 1 in 5000 to 1,000,000.[15,16] After the first 4 mL, essentially zero osteoprogenitor cells were found in the aspirate.[17]

Finally, another newer source of autogenous graft is the medullary canals of the femur and tibia, using the reamer irrigator aspirator. This subject is discussed in detail in articles found elsewhere in this issue.

DONOR SITES

The iliac crest has been and is still the most common area for obtaining autogenous cancellous bone graft because of the relative ease of access and the quantity of graft that may be obtained without compromising bone integrity to skeletal support. Iliac crest bone graft also contains all elements recommended for bone graft: osteogenic cells, an osteoconductive scaffold, and osteoinductive proteins. Graft may be obtained from the posterior or anterior ilium,

a decision generally determined by patient positioning: posterior grafts are obtained when the patient is prone, whereas the anterior approach is used with the patient supine. Harvesting of the graft is accomplished by opening a cortical window and removing cancellous bone. Studies have reported volumes of around 50 mL from anterior and posterior sites.

When using the posterior ilium, the posterior superior iliac spine is palpated and an incision is made centered around this structure, being mindful to not extend beyond 8 cm from the posterior superior iliac spine, where the cluneal nerves are at risk. Additionally, the ligamentous structures of the sacroiliac joint (medial) and the sciatic foramen (distal) should be avoided to prevent sacroiliac instability or damage to the sciatic nerve and the superior gluteal artery. Approaching anteriorly, the incision should extend along the anterior ilium, stopping 1 to 2 cm lateral to the anterior superior iliac spine to avoid the lateral femoral cutaneous nerve and inguinal ligament.[18]

Although generally regarded as safe, complications and morbidity associated with iliac crest bone grafting have been reported, mostly with anterior crest harvest sites. Wound complications can occur in approximately 21% of these grafts when incisions are made directly over the crest, but far fewer when the incision is made superior or inferior to the crest.[19] Nerve injury can occur to the lateral femoral cutaneous nerve, which has a variable course but most frequently exits anterior and inferior to the anterior superior iliac spine.

Although anesthesia from transaction of the lateral femoral cutaneous nerve is minimal and well tolerated, painful neuromas can result in a condition called *meralgia paresthetica*. The authors believe that in pelvic and acetabular surgery, it is better to surgically transect the nerve rather than risk a stretch injury, which could lead to meralgia paresthetica.

Blood loss is also expected with iliac crest bone grafting. Arterial injury and hemorrhage is rare, although reported with posterior grafting and violation of the sciatic notch. Hematoma formation, which has been described in as high as 4% to 10% of patients, can be decreased with topical hemostatic agents, and suction drainage.[7] The hematoma and any subsequent drainage can also rarely lead to infection. Arteriovenous fistula and ureteral injury can occur with posterior iliac crest harvesting, although these are limited to case reports.[20] Less commonly, gluteal gait from abductor weakness can occur from excessive stripping of the outer table.

Pain is probably the most common complaint after iliac crest bone grafting. Laurie[19] reported that all patients had moderate pain at 6 weeks, and 10% experienced pain beyond 2 years. Goulet and colleagues[21] found 38% had pain extending to 6 months and 18% experienced pain at 2 years postoperatively.

Unfortunately, although most pain seems to fade with time, chronic pain is likely an unavoidable result in a small percentage of patients.[22] Because some reports indicate that the incidence of pain may be less than the 38% reported by Goulet and colleagues,[21] some technical factors may be associated with this particular morbidity, and attention to surgical technique and soft tissue handling may minimize this morbidity.

The authors have found that when significant lengths of crest have been harvested (as in tricortical grafts), reconstructing the arc of the iliac wing is helpful to prevent muscle herniation and painful belt wear. Many techniques and products exist for this purpose, but the authors have found that use of a curved 3.5-mm pelvic reconstruction plate across the gap is helpful and, unless incompetence of the iliacus muscle is present, visceral herniation is rare. Still, this complication is rare and serious, as shown in (**Fig. 5**).

In an attempt to avoid the morbidity of iliac crest harvesting, other sites and techniques have been developed. Westrich and colleagues[23] described a method of harvesting using an acetabular corticocancellous reamer, which they found to be safe and efficacious compared with traditional methods. They note an advantage in the amount of graft obtained (three reamer cups full), but fail to provide a defined quantity.

Sanders and DiPasquale[24] described a similar technique using an acetabular reamer, but in the posterior pelvis. Similarly, copious amounts of graft are reported to be available but not quantified. These investigators reported less discomfort while obtaining large amounts of graft.

The tibia and distal femur have been described as a site for obtaining autogenous cancellous bone graft. The distal tibia is commonly used in foot and ankle surgery because of the proximity to the surgical site and also because small amounts of graft are needed in these procedures. in 1991. O'Keeffe[25] described the proximal tibial metaphysis as an alternative to the iliac crest. Reports have shown that up to 30 mL of graft can be obtained from the proximal tibial metaphysis.[26] Krause and Perry[27] proposed the distal femur as a graft site, providing an average quantity of 10.4 g. They also acknowledge the devastating potential of a supracondylar femur fracture, but note that with a 6-week non-weightbearing period, patients experienced no major complications.

RECIPIENT SITES

In the forearm, Wright and colleagues[28] retrospectively investigated the acute cancellous bone grafting in radius and ulna fractures. They found union rates to be comparable in grafted and ungrafted individuals treated with open reduction and internal fixation. They concluded that routine use of bone grafting in comminuted forearm fractures is not indicated. Wei and colleagues[29] similarly studied bone grafting of acute forearm fractures. They also found no significant difference in union rate in groups treated with or without cancellous grafting. Neither study investigated significant bone loss, which is uncommon in the forearm.

Ring and colleagues[30] presented a group of patients who had diaphyseal forearm nonunions and segmental defects that were treated with plate fixation and autogenous cancellous grafting. Without a control group, they found that all 35 patients healed within 6 months without subsequent procedures and that they experienced an improvement in upper extremity function.

Barbieri and colleagues[31] reported on the technique of iliac crest bone block grafting to treat forearm nonunions associated with diaphyseal defects in 12 patients. The graft incorporated without additional procedures in 10 of 12 patients.

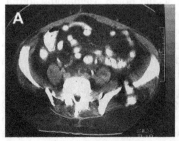 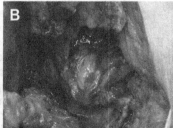 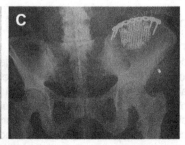

Fig. 5. (A) CT scan of a patient who presented after colonic herniation through the iliac wing after an aggressive bone graft procedure. (B) Intraoperative photo of the patient showing colonic viscera through the iliac wing. (C) Radiograph showing the reconstruction with retention screen and reconstruction plate.

The investigators concluded that the technique of bone block grafting to correct diaphyseal defects of the radius or ulna is relatively easy to perform and has a high success rate.

Similar to the forearm, albeit to a greater extent, the humerus has a very good soft tissue envelope. Although no literature is available on the acute bone grafting of humerus fractures, its use in nonunions is well established. Hierholzer reported the results of treating humeral nonunion or delayed union with open reduction and internal fixation combined with either iliac crest autograft or demineralized bone matrix grafting. Union was achieved in 100% of patients treated with autograft and 97% treated with demineralized bone matrix grafting. The study did not find significant morbidity associated with harvesting at the donor site.[32]

Hsu and colleagues[33] performed a retrospective review of 105 humeral nonunions over 19 years treated with compression plating and autogenous cancellous bone grafting. They found all fractures to have united at an average of 16 weeks, concluding that this treatment option was reliable and effective in humeral nonunion.

The femur has one of the best healing rates in the body, and no studies analyze the use of acute autogenous bone graft in fractures. Correspondingly, the literature on femoral nonunions is sparse and often involves small sample sizes. In the supracondylar region, Chapman and Finkemeier[34] reported excellent union rates with revision open reduction, internal fixation, and autogenous cancellous grafting, with all 18 fractures going on to union. Wang and Weng[35] combined autogenous bone grafting with allograft struts and also achieved union in all 13 patients in their study. The preservation of blood supply using proper surgical technique was stressed in these studies.

Finkemeier and Chapman[36] reviewed a series of patients who had femoral diaphyseal nonunions. Before bone grafting a diaphyseal nonunion, they recommended a reamed exchange nailing, reserving autogenous bone grafting as a second-stage procedure.

The tibia remains one of the most grafted sites in the body for various reasons. It is the most commonly fractured long bone, has a relatively poor soft tissue envelope and vascular supply (especially distally), and is frequently devascularized and contaminated when associated with high-energy open injuries. Many studies have investigated acute bone grafting of tibial fractures; however, because many severe tibia fractures require soft tissue reconstruction, such as free or rotational flaps, the grafting is typically delayed. Once soft tissues have healed, which often occurs

in 6 to 8 weeks, the bed is appropriate for bone grafting.

Blick and colleagues[37] investigated the use of prophylactic bone grafting in 53 high-energy tibial fractures over a 2-year period. The patients were matched with historical controls that required bone grafting after a diagnosis of delayed union or nonunion. Patients underwent planned posterolateral cancellous bone grafting on all fractures in the study within 16 weeks. The investigators found a statistically significant difference in time to union between the groups. They recommend posterolateral grafting at 2 weeks in open fractures closed secondarily or those needing only a rotational flap for coverage. In wounds requiring free flaps for coverage, they recommend bone grafting at 6 weeks.

Christian and colleagues[38] analyzed the use of massive amounts of autogenous bone graft in the treatment of open tibial fractures with large diaphyseal defects. Eight patients with grade 3B open tibial fractures were treated with external fixation, soft tissue coverage, and antibiotic bead placement initially. At a planned later date, the beads were removed and a large iliac crest autogenous graft was placed 6 to 8 weeks after coverage of the wound. The fractures healed in all eight patients. The authors note that this option is an alternative to free vascularized fibular graft (FVFG) in patients who have either a single vessel to the leg (and therefore are not candidates for microvascular anastomosis) or wounds worrisome for possible infection. They comment that failed FVFG is more likely to result in amputation, whereas their method provides for easier further attempts at limb salvage.

In a review of management of open grade III tibial shaft fractures, Burgess and colleagues[39] agreed with planned autogenous bone grafting once the soft tissue envelope heals at approximately 4 to 6 weeks. They note that FVFG may be used for large defects but did not specify when this may be most useful.

Yaremchuk and colleagues[40] used a similar protocol for treating osteocutaneous injuries to the leg. They performed scheduled bone grafting once soft tissue wounds were healed at a range of 6 to 16 weeks. Cancellous grafting was performed for defects smaller than 8 cm, and FVFG for those larger than 8 cm. However, the investigators note that the free muscle flap provides an excellent blood supply for bone graft incorporation, and that cancellous grafts may be effective in gaps larger than 8 cm.

In a review of management strategies for tibial bone loss, Watson and colleagues[41] analyzed 50 fractures of the tibia with greater than 50%

circumferential bone loss. Cancellous bone grafting was performed in 37 of these patients with good results. The investigators comment that posterolateral bone grafting in these severe injuries can be technically challenging because of disruption or scarring along the interosseous membrane, posing a risk to the neurovascular structures.

In the presence of a free muscle transfer for coverage, the anterolateral approach is easier and safer, and a large, well-covered pocket for graft placement is often present. Another theoretical concern with acute bone grafting is the possibility of graft resorption during the acute healing period, which is often an inflammatory phase. The placement of autogenous graft into an inflammatory tissue bed may result in a resorptive response, which would waste precious autograft.

Furthermore, in open injuries, the risk for infection and graft wastage is also a significant concern. For that reason, some investigators have advocated using allograft and demineralized bone matrix, with or without marrow aspirate, for early grafting with no risk for autograft wastage. Unfortunately, the results of this technique have not been well validated with high-level scientific studies.[42]

The most common condition for tibial grafting remains the tibial nonunion. Bone grafting for tibial nonunion has been described dating back to the early 1900s. Anterolateral grafting was used commonly in the past, but fell out of favor because of poor soft tissue envelope and small area for graft placement. Harmon[7] advocated posterolateral bone grafting of the tibia, which remains the gold standard for treating midshaft and distal tibial nonunion. However, because of the nearby neurovascular structures in the proximal one third of the tibia, the posteromedial approach to bone grafting has been recommended.[43]

From the 1950s through the 1970s, numerous reports discussed the use and location of bone grafting in treating tibial nonunion. In 1955, Jones and Barnett[44] proclaimed success with posterolateral bone grafting of infected tibial nonunions without resecting the fibrous union, and often without treating the infection. In 1966, Hanson and Eppright[45] reported on a similar series with good results. Blair[46] described the use of a diamond-shaped graft wedged between the tibial nonunion site. His idea was novel in that it lacked placement of additional hardware into the wound, although further studies surrounding this technique are lacking.

In 1982, Gershuni and Pinsker[47] analyzed 40 tibial nonunions treated with autograft and cast immobilization. Although they achieved a union rate of 85%, they also experienced significant angular deformity. They recommend treatment with stable internal or external fixation (rather than cast immobilization) because of similar union rates and better functional results. In 1980, Reckling and Waters[48] reported on a large series of tibial nonunions treated with posterolateral corticocancellous bone grafting. They claim that this is a single nondestructive procedure with a high degree of success because the graft is vascularized quickly. They also claim that union can occur in the setting of infection with cessation of the drainage on union.

In 1990, Meister and colleagues[49] reported on 12 years of treating tibial nonunions and delayed unions with autogenous grafting, reaffirming that it is the most effective and reliable treatment available. Simpson and colleagues[50] also reported in 1990 on 30 high-energy tibial nonunions with a 97% union rate after posterolateral autogenous bone grafting, and concluded that "posterolateral bone grafts consistently produced rapid healing of delayed union as well as established nonunion." Similarly in 1992, Simon and colleagues[51] reported good results with 62 tibial nonunions over an 18-year period treated with posterolateral bone grafting using solid iliac crest, nonvascularized fibula, and cancellous iliac crest. As their treatment algorithm changed over the analyzed period, they used different graft types. They concluded that "cortico-cancellous bone chips resulted in a shorter healing time compared with a nonvascularized fibular graft or a massive corticocancellous bone block."

In a 1996 review article on tibial nonunion treatment options, Wiss and Stetson[52] commented that autogenous cancellous grafts remained the gold standard in the treatment of tibial nonunion and can be used to treat segments as large as 6 cm with successful outcome in 88% to 95% of cases. Recently, Ryzewicz and colleagues[53] reported on the use of "central bone grafting" for tibial nonunion. This technique involves a lateral approach, anterior to the fibula, and creation of a tibiofibular synostosis. The investigators claim that compared with the standard posterolateral bone grafting, this technique has decreased risk to the neurovascular bundle, the surgical dissection is easier, and the patient can be positioned supine.

VASCULARIZED OSSEOUS GRAFTS

In defects greater than 6–8 cm, vascularized grafts have been proposed to have significant advantages over conventional grafts.[54] FVFGs were first described in the late 1970s by Ian Taylor,[55] who transferred a segment of fibula to the contralateral tibia. The FVFG can be transferred in several configurations and in varying compositions, including skin, fascia, muscle, or physis.[56,57] It is indicated in skeletal defects greater than 5 to 6 cm or those associated with poor vascularity. The FVFG is taken as a pedicle with the peroneal artery, which arises from the posterior tibial artery, 3 to 4 cm distal to its bifurcation into the anterior and posterior tibial arteries.[58] The peroneal artery is typically the least dominant of the three arteries supplying the lower extremity and can be sacrificed in these situations.

However, in an analysis of leg angiographies before FVFG, Lutz and colleagues[59] noted a single case of the peroneal artery being the dominant artery to the leg. This finding was associated with an abnormal pedal pulse. Therefore, in the context of abnormal pulses or with previous lower extremity trauma, angiography should be performed before proceeding with any surgical intervention to lessen the risk for an iatrogenic dysvascular leg.

After implantation, the graft should be monitored for viability (acutely), union (intermediately), and hypertrophy (late).[20] One of the major disadvantages of the FVFG is the potential for late fracture. Because the fibula has a smaller cross-sectional area than the native tibia, repetitive full load weightbearing may result in an overloading and subsequent fatigue/stress fracture in up to one third of lower extremity cases. Therefore, protected weightbearing is recommended until adequate hypertrophy of the incorporated fibular graft occurs. Unfortunately, this may take several years and diminishes the attractiveness of this technique compared with distraction osteogenesis. Watson and colleagues[41] abandoned the use of FVFG for tibial bone loss because of the reliability of current bone transport techniques.

Cove and colleagues[60] retrospectively reported on a series of 44 patients who had femoral diaphyseal nonunions. All patients (except one) underwent autogenous cancellous grafting, and eight patients also had an FVFG. Various fixation methods were used. Several patients had difficult infections before intervention, but good results were reported.

In 1995, Doi and colleagues[61] reported on 26 patients who had bone loss or infected nonunion treated with single-stage debridement and osteocutaneous FVFG. Union and eradication of infection was achieved in 25 of 26 patients; however, graft hypertrophy was not sufficient for weightbearing until 18 months.

The most common complication with FVFG is muscle weakness, usually transient, of the flexor hallucis longus, extensor hallucis longus, or peroneal muscles.[62] Ankle instability has also been reported, and to avoid destabilization of the syndesmosis distally, approximately 6 cm of distal fibula should be preserved.

In contrast with lower extremity applications, FVFGs in the upper extremity have had better results. Adani and colleagues[63] report on a series of 12 patients who had segmental defects of the forearm treated with FVFG. Plate fixation was used in 10, and external fixation in the remaining 2. Union was achieved in 11 of 12 patients. The investigators recommend the vascularized fibular in patients who have intractable nonunions that have failed to respond to conventional bone grafting or who have large bone defects (>6 cm).

Adani and colleagues[64] also reported on a series of 13 patients who had humeral nonunions with an average defect of 10.5 cm. They performed FVFG with a mean healing time of 6 months. Among these patients, 9 healed primarily after the procedure, 3 required additional bone grafting, and 1 required a second FVFG. They recommend FVFG in patients who have a chronic nonunion with bone atrophy, and after sufficient debridement in the setting of infection.

Jupiter and colleagues[65] reported on a series of patients who had radius nonunions from segmental loss and soft tissue loss. They performed FVFG with combined septocutaneous flap on nine patients with good results. However, this option may be one of very few possibilities in patients who have severe bone and soft tissue loss. Beredjiklian and colleagues[66] reported on five patients who had chronic distal humeral nonunions, with good results, concluding that this is a viable procedure, especially in younger patients in whom arthroplasty is not an option.

Solid iliac crest bone graft may also be obtained as a vascular graft, and may be taken alone or as an osteocutaneous flap. It is harvested as a pedicle with the deep circumflex iliac artery and vein. This procedure is performed through a generous incision along the anterior iliac crest. Entering the inguinal canal, the origin of the deep circumflex iliac artery is identified as it branches off the lateral aspect of the external iliac artery, and traced to the anterior superior iliac spine (also note that the superficial circumflex iliac may also be harvested in the case of an osteocutaneous flap).

Vascularized iliac crest grafts may perform better than FVFG in end-to-end bone healing because of the exposure to cancellous bone. Additionally, the iliac graft is preferred in patients requiring contouring of the graft and skin surface.[67] Proponents of the FVFG would comment that because of its curvature, shape, and limited size, the iliac crest is more difficult to use than the vascularized fibula. Vascularized rib grafts have been described more frequently in plastic surgery literature. They are allegorically referred to as the "Eve" procedure. Both single and double rib transfers have been described. The graft is harvested as a pedicle to the serratus and has been generally limited to treatment of clavicle nonunions.[68]

SUMMARY

Solid and cancellous autogenous bone grafts are well described for fractures with bone loss and nonunions. The iliac crest remains the main location for harvest, and the tibia the main recipient site, but the morbidity of the procedure remains significant. Newer harvesting methods and alternative autogenous donor sites are being investigated and could potentially alleviate the need for pelvic autograft. Autogenous grafting for the upper extremity is less common, because other modalities have proven successful and do not incur the morbidity of autograft. However, in larger defects of the upper extremity, FVFGs have been shown to be successful, but their use is potentially problematic in the lower extremity. Distraction osteogenesis remains the best alternative in massive limb reconstructions.

REFERENCES

1. Weiss LE. Web watch. Tissue Eng 2002;8(1):167.
2. Bone Grafts. A US Market Report. Global Industry Analysts 2009:1–353.
3. Ollier L. Traite de la regeneration des os. Mason, Paris, 1867 [in French].
4. Phemister DB. The fate of transplanted bone and regenerative power of its various constituents. Surg Gynecol Obstet 1914;19:303–33.
5. Phemister DB. Treatment of ununited fractures by onlay bone grafts without screw or tie fixation and without breaking down of the fibrous union. J Bone Joint Surg Am 1947;29(4):946–60.
6. Judet R, Judet J. Osteo-periosteal decortication. Principle, technique, indications and results. Mem Acad Chir 1965;91(15):463–70.
7. Harmon PH. A simplified surgical approach to the posterior tibia for bone-grafting and fibular transference. J Bone Joint Surg Am 1945;47:179–90.
8. Urist MR. Bone: formation by autoinduction. Science 1965;150:893–9.
9. Urist MR, Strates BS. Bone morphogenetic protein. J Dent Res 1971;50(6):1392–406.
10. Einhorn TA, O'Keefe RJ, Buckwalker JA, editors. Orthopaedic basic science: foundations of clinical practice. 3rd edition. Rosemont: American Academy of Orthopaedic Surgeons, 2007.
11. Rodringo J, Chapman MW. Bone grafting, bone graft substitutes, and growth factors. In: Chapman MW, Szabo RM, Marder RA, et al., editors. Chapman's orthopedic surgery. 3rd edition. Philadelphia: Lippincott Williams & Wilkins 2001. p. 181–211.
12. Ilizarov GA. Basic principles of transosseous compression and distraction osteosynthesis. Ortop Travmatol Protez 1971;32(11):7–15.
13. Connolly JF. Clinical use of marrow osteoprogenitor cells to stimulate osteogenesis. Clin Orthop Relat Res 1998;355:S257–66.
14. Wilkins RM, Chimenti BT, Rifkin RM. Percutaneous treatment of long bone nonunions: the use of autologous bone marrow and allograft bone matrix. Orthopedics 2003;26(5):S549–54.
15. Bidula J, Boehm C, Powell K, et al. Osteogenic progenitors in bone marrow aspirates from smokers and nonsmokers. Clin Orthop Relat Res 2006;442:252–9.
16. Muschler GF, Nitto H, Boehm C, et al. Age- and gender-related changes in the cellularity of human bone marrow and the prevalence of osteoblastic progenitors. J Orthop Res 2001;19(1):117–25.
17. Muschler GF, Boehm C, Easley K. Aspiration to obtain osteoblast progenitor cells from human bone marrow: the influence of aspiration volume. J Bone Joint Surg Am 1997;79(11):1699–709.
18. Kurz LT, Garfin SR, Booth RE Jr. Harvesting autogenous iliac bone grafts: a review of complications and techniques. Spine 1989;14(12):1324–31.
19. Laurie SWS, Kaban LB, Mulliken JB, et al. Donor site morbidity after harvesting rib and iliac bone. Plast Reconstr Surg 1984;73(6):933–8.
20. Escalas F, DeWald RL. Combined traumatic arteriovenous fistula and ureteral injury: a complication of iliac bone-grafting. J Bone Joint Surg Am 1977;59(2):270–1.
21. Goulet JA, Senunas LE, DeSilva GL, et al. Autogenous iliac crest bone graft: complications and functional assessment. Clin Orthop Relat Res 1997;339:76–81.
22. Younger EM, Chapman MW. Morbidity at bone graft donor sites. J Orthop Trauma 1989;3(3):192–5.
23. Westrich GH, Geller DS, O'Malley MJ, et al. Anterior iliac crest bone graft harvesting using the corticancellous reamer system. J Orthop Trauma 2001;15(7):500–6.
24. Sanders R, DiPasquale T. A technique for obtaining bone graft. J Orthop Trauma 1989;3(4):287–9.
25. O'Keeffe RM Jr, Reimer BL, Butterfield SL. Harvesting of autogenous cancellous bone graft from the proximal tibial metaphysis. A review of 230 cases. J Orthop Trauma 1991;5(4):469–74.
26. Geideman W, Early JS, Brodsky J. Clinical results of harvesting autogenous graft from the ipsilateral

proximal tibia for use in foot and ankle surgery. Foot Ankle Int 2004;25(7):451–5.

27. Krause JO, Perry CR. Distal femur as a donor site of autogenous cancellous bone graft. J Orthop Trauma 1995;9(2):145–51.

28. Wright RR, Schmeling GJ, Schwab JP. The necessity of acute bone grafting in diaphyseal forearm fractures: a retrospective review. J Orthop Trauma 1997;11(4):288–94.

29. Wei SY, Born CT, Abene A, et al. Diaphyseal forearm fractures treated with and without bone graft. J Trauma 1999;46(6):1045–8.

30. Ring D, Allende C, Jafarnia K, et al. Ununited diaphyseal forearm fractures with segmental defects: plate fixation and autogenous cancellous bone-grafting. J Bone Joint Surg Am 2004; 86(11):2440–5.

31. Barbieri CH, Mazzer N, Aranda CA, et al. Use of a bone block graft from the iliac crest with rigid fixation to correct diaphyseal defects of the radius and ulna. J Hand Surg Br 1997;22(3):395–401.

32. Hierholzer C, Sama D, Toro JB, et al. Plate fixation of ununited humeral shaft fractures: effect of type of bone graft on healing. J Bone Joint Surg Am 2006; 88(7):1442–7.

33. Hsu TL, Chiu FY, Chen CM, et al. Treatment of nonunion of humeral shaft fracture with dynamic compression plate and cancellous bone graft. J Chin Med Assoc 2005;68(2):73–6.

34. Chapman MW, Finkemeier CG. Treatment of supracondylar nonunion of the femur with plate fixation and bone graft. J Bone Joint Surg Am 1999;81(9): 1217–28.

35. Wang JW, Weng LH. Treatment of distal femoral nonunion with internal fixation, cortical allograft struts, and autogenous bone-grafting. J Bone Joint Surg Am 2003;85(3):436–40.

36. Finkemeier CG, Chapman MW. Treatment of femoral diaphyseal nonunions. Clin Orthop Relat Res 2002; 398:223–34.

37. Blick SS, Brumback RJ, Lakatos R, et al. Early prophylactic bone grafting of high-energy tibial fractures. Clin Orthop Relat Res 1989;240:21–41.

38. Christian EP, Bosse MJ, Robb G. Reconstruction of large diaphyseal defects, without free fibular transfer, in grade-IIIB tibial fractures. J Bone Joint Surg Am 1989;71(7):994–1004.

39. Burgess AR, Poka A, Brumback RJ, et al. Management of open grade III tibial fractures. Orthop Clin North Am 1987;18(1):85–93.

40. Yaremchuk MJ, Brumback RJ, Manson PN, et al. Acute and definitive management of traumatic osteocutaneous defects of the lower extremity. Plast Reconstr Surg 1987;80(1):1–14.

41. Watson JT, Anders M, Moed BR. Management strategies for bone loss in tibial shaft fractures. Clin Orthop Relat Res 1995;315:138–52.

42. Ziran BH, Smith WR, Morgan SJ. Use of calcium-based demineralized bone matrix/allograft for nonunions and posttraumatic reconstruction of the appendicular skeleton: preliminary results and complications. J Trauma 2007;63(6):1324–8.

43. DeCoster TA, Gehlert RJ, Mikola EA, et al. Management of posttraumatic segmental bone defects. J Am Acad Orthop Surg 2004;12(1):28–38.

44. Jones KG, Barnett HC. Cancellous bone grafting for non-union of the tibia through the posterolateral approach. J Bone Joint Surg Am 1955;27(6): 1250–9.

45. Hanson LW, Eppright RH. Posterior bone grafting of the tibial for nonunion. J Bone Joint Surg Am 1966; 48:27.

46. Blair HC. A diamond shaped graft from the ilium for nonunion of the tibia. J Bone Joint Surg Am 1951; 33(2):362–7.

47. Gershuni DH, Pinsker R. Bone grafting for nonunion of fractures of the tibia: a critical review. J Trauma 1982;22(1):43–9.

48. Reckling FW, Waters CH. Treatment of non-unions of fractures of the tibial diaphysis by posterolateral cortical cancellous bone-grafting. J Bone Joint Surg Am 1980;62(6):936–41.

49. Meister K, Segal D, Whitelaw GP. The role of bone grafting in the treatment of delayed unions and nonunions of the tibia. Orthop Rev 1990;19(3): 260–71.

50. Simpson JM, Ebraheim NA, An HS, et al. Posterolateral bone graft of the tibia. Clin Orthop Relat Res 1990;251:200–6.

51. Simon JP, Stuyck J, Hoogmartens M, et al. Posterolateral bone grafting for nonunion of the tibia. Acta Orthop Belg 1992;58(3):308–13.

52. Wiss DA, Stetson WB. Tibial nonunion: treatment alternatives. J Am Acad Orthop Surg 1996;4:249–57.

53. Ryzewicz M, Morgan SJ, Linford E, et al. Central bone grafting for nonunion of fractures of the tibia: a retrospective series. J Bone Joint Surg Br 2009; 91(4):522–9.

54. Weiland AJ, Moore JR, Daniel RK. Vascularized bone autografts: experience with 41 cases. Clin Orthop Relat Res 1983;174:87–95.

55. Taylor GI, Miller GD, Ham FJ. The free vascularized bone graft. A clinical extension of microvascular techniques. Plast Reconstr Surg 1975;55(5): 533–44.

56. Innocenti M, Ceruso M, Manfrini M, et al. Free vascularized growth-plate transfer after bone tumor resection in children. J Reconstr Microsurg 1998;14(2): 137–43.

57. Wood MB. Free vascularized fibula grafting—25 years experience: tips, techniques, and pearls. Orthop Clin North Am 2007;38(1):1–12.

58. Malizos KN, Zalavras CG, Soucacos PN, et al. Free vascularized fibular grafts for reconstruction of

skeletal defects. J Am Acad Orthop Surg 2004; 12(5):360–9.

59. Lutz BS, Wei FC, Ng SH, et al. Routine donor leg angiography before vascularized free fibula transplantation is not necessary: a prospective study in 120 clinical cases. Plast Reconstr Surg 1999; 103(1):121–7.

60. Cove JA, Lhowe DW, Jupiter JB, et al. The management of femoral diaphyseal nonunions. J Orthop Trauma 1997;11(7):513–20.

61. Doi K, Kawakami F, Hiura Y, et al. One-stage treatment of infected bone defects of the tibia with skin loss by free vascularized osteocutaneous grafts. Microsurgery 1995;16(10):704–12.

62. Vail TP, Urbaniak JR. Donor site morbidity with use of vascularized autogenous fibular grafts. J Bone Joint Surg Am 1996;78(2):204–11.

63. Adani R, Delbroix L, Innocenti M, et al. Reconstruction of large posttraumatic skeletal defects of the forearm by vascularized free fibular graft. Microsurgery 2004;24(6):423–9.

64. Adani R, Delcroix L, Tarallo L, et al. Reconstruction of posttraumatic bone defects of the humerus with vascularized fibular graft. J Shoulder Elbow Surg 2008;17(4):578–84.

65. Jupiter JB, Gerhard HJ, Guerrero J, et al. Treatment of segmental defects of the radius with use of the vascularized osteoseptocutaneous fibular autogenous graft. J Bone Joint Surg Am 1997;79(4): 542–50.

66. Beredjiklian PK, Hotchkiss RN, Athanasian EA, et al. Recalcitrant nonunion of the distal humerus: treatment with free vascularized bone grafting. Clin Orthop Relat Res 2005;435:134–9.

67. Salibian AH, Anzel SH, Salyer WA. Transfer of vascularized grafts of iliac bone to the extremities. J Bone Joint Surg Am 1987;69(9):1319–27.

68. Werner CM, Favre P, van Lenthe HG, et al. Pedicled vascularized rib transfer for reconstruction of clavicle nonunions with bony defects: anatomical and biomechanical considerations. Plast Reconstr Surg 2007;120(1):173–80.

The Concept of Induced Membrane for Reconstruction of Long Bone Defects

Alain C. Masquelet, MD*, Thierry Begue, MD

KEYWORDS

- Bone reconstruction • Bone defect • Membrane
- Osteoinductive factors • Bone healing

The reconstruction of wide long bone diaphyseal defects is often the major challenge in limb salvage whatever the etiology of bone loss. The most common and widely accepted procedures are the vascularized bone free transfer and the Ilizarov bone transport method. Bone autograft is not advocated when the defect is over 4 to 5 cm. When diaphyseal defects larger than 6 cm are reconstructed with autologous bone graft, healing is incomplete because of graft resorption even in a good vascularized muscular envelope.[1,2] Experimental study and clinical experience concerning osteoperiosteal flaps were encouraging,[3] but the limited sizes of harvested flaps on the human body incited the authors to abandon this technique of bone reconstruction

Since 1986, the authors' routinely use a technique that has permitted the authors to elaborate the concept of induced membrane and to reconstruct large defects with nonvascularized bone autograft.[4,5] Induced membrane is different from the bioresorbable polylactide membranes experimentally tested to treat critical size, segmental defects in rabbits[6] or sheep.[7,8]

The aim of this article is to present the membrane as a biological model, to compare the results of two clinical series, and to discuss the implications of the model.

PRINCIPLES OF TECHNIQUE

The reconstruction needs to have two different operative stages (**Fig. 1**). The first stage is comprised of a radical debridement, a soft-tissue repair by flaps when needed, and the insertion of a polymethyl methacrylate (PMMA) cement spacer into the bone defect. The second stage is performed 6 to 8 weeks later, when the definitive healing of soft tissue is acquired. The spacer is removed, but the membrane that is induced by the cement is left in place **Fig. 1**A. The cavity is filled up by morcellized cancellous bone autograft harvested from the iliac crests **Fig. 1**B. Sometimes, when the amount of autograft is not sufficient or to spare an iliac crest, bone substitute (demineralized ox bone) is added to the cancellous bone according to a ratio that is not over 1:3.

Several technical details should be emphasized. At the first stage, the cement must be wrapped around the bone extremities to allow detaching small pieces of the ends of the bone and lifting it with a bit of the induced membrane, at the second stage. When the bone graft is placed into the tube, the soft tissues, including the membrane, are sutured close to the graft resulting in a containment system **Fig. 1**C. When treating a diaphyseal defect of the tibia, the cement is applied on the fibula as far as possible to obtain a very strong reconstruction. Moreover, at the second stage, the authors routinely perform an intertibiofibular graft at both extremities of the tibial defect, by a posterior approach **Fig. 1**D. In reconstruction of the lower limb, the full weight bearing is usually authorized to patients at 5 to 6 months with the protection of the external fixator. Then the fixation is dynamized during 1 month and

Department of Orthopedic and Traumatology, Avicenne Hospital, Medical University of Paris, 125, route de Stalingrad, 93009 Bobigny, Paris, France
* Corresponding author.
E-mail address: alain-charles.masquelet@avc.aphp.fr (A.C. Masquelet).

Orthop Clin N Am 41 (2010) 27–37
doi:10.1016/j.ocl.2009.07.011
0030-5898/09/$ – see front matter © 2010 Published by Elsevier Inc.

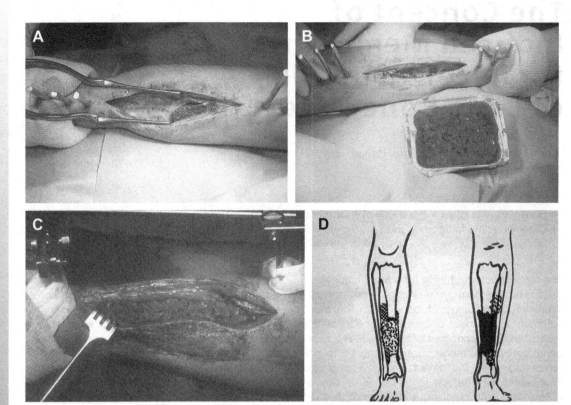

Fig. 1. Elements of technique. (*A*). The preoperative aspect of the membrane just before filling up the cavity Note the petaling of the bone extremity. (*B*) Morcellized cancellous bone graft; the chips should be as small as possible. The alveolar structure of the cancellous bone permits a fast revascularization by the vascular buds issued from the membrane. (*C*) The cavity is filled up; the suture en bloc of the membrane and subcutaneous tissue results in a containment system. (*D*) Principles of reconstruction of the tibia. At the first stage the PMMA spacer is applied on the fibula. At the time of reconstruction an intertibiofibular graft is performed on both extremities.

finally removed 1 month later. In 1990, the surprising results of the authors' first cases incited them to undertake experimental and fundamental studies to elucidate the role of the membrane induced by the cement spacer. One of the main interrogations concerned the absence of resorption of the autograft.

The Foreign Body-induced Membrane

Initially, the role of the cement spacer was to avoid the collapse of the soft tissue into the bone defect and to prepare the bone reconstruction. Moreover, as most of the authors' clinical cases were post-traumatic septic nonunions, the spacer was considered an excellent witness of successful debridement in the absence of recurrent infection after 2 months. The initial reason for which the authors' did not excise the membrane was to prevent excessive bleeding. Finally, the main role of the cement is biological, by inducing a foreign-body surrounding membrane.

The first step of the investigation was to confirm the role of the membrane. Experimental study was done at the AO Development Institute of Davos[9]

and it was asserted that the membrane avoided the resorption of the cancellous bone and had a positive effect upon the healing of the autograft. Material comprised 30 sheep on which a segmental femoral defect, 3 cm in length, was created, filled up with a PMMA cement spacer, and stabilized with a plate. One month later, four groups were constituted after removing the spacer:

- Group A: the membrane was maintained and filled up with cancellous bone chips.
- Group B: the membrane was excised and the defect was filled up with cancellous bone chips.
- Group C: the membrane alone was maintained without filling.
- Group D: the membrane was excised and the defect was not filled up.

As expected, no bone formation was noted in groups C and D. In group B, bone healing was partially obtained with an important resorption in all cases. In group A, bone healing was acquired without reduction of the volume of the initial graft.

The second step of the investigation was to precise the role of the membrane by evaluating its histologic and biochemical characteristics.[10] Histologic and immunochemistry studies were performed and the following data have been established:

- The membrane is richly vascularized in all its layers.
- The inner part (face to the cement) is a synovial like epithelium and the outer part is made of fibroblasts, myofibroblasts, and collagen.

- The membrane secretes growth factors: high concentration of VEGF and TGF Beta 1 were observed as early as the second week. BMP-2 is at its highest level at the fourth week.

Finally, membrane extracts stimulated bone marrow cell proliferation and differentiation to osteoblastic lineage.

Clinical experience showed that the cancellous bone inside the membrane is not submitted to resorption. As shown by a case report,[11] after healing, macroscopic examination of transverse

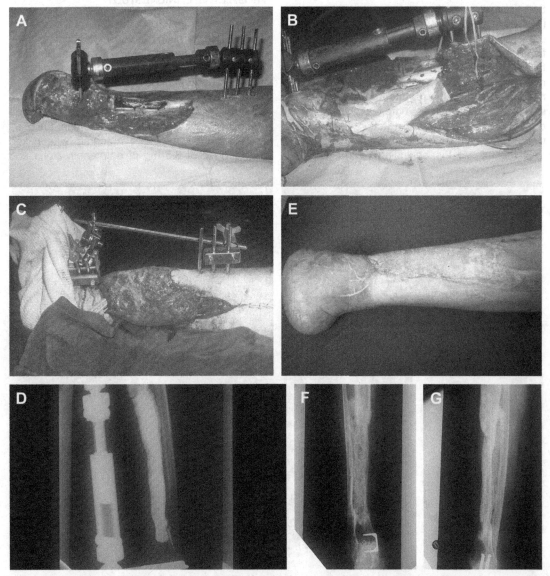

Fig. 2. Infected nonunion of the leg in a 27-year-old woman. The fore foot was amputated but the stump was sensible. (A) Initial aspect. (B) Radical debridement and preparation of the proximal vessels for covering with a free flap. (C) Latissimus dorsi in place. (D) The cement spacer under the muscle flap. Defect was 18 cm length. (E) Final clinical result. (F, G) Radiologic aspect 1 year later. Full weight bearing was permitted at the end of 6th month.

section of the healed bone graft exhibits normal bone anatomy, and the junction between the normal bone and the graft was difficult to see by macroscopic examination of longitudinal sections.

RETROSPECTIVE CLINICAL EXPERIENCE

Between 1986 and 1999,[4] the authors did a series of 35 reconstructions of long bone segmental defects ranging from 5 to 24 cm after debridement. Lower limb was involved in 29 cases and the majority of cases were posttraumatic septic nonunions of the leg (23 cases) (**Figs. 2** and **3**). Upper limb was concerned in six cases (**Fig. 4**). Soft-tissue repair by flaps was needed in 28 cases (14 free flaps and 14 pedicled flaps). Immediate complications concerned the failure of the free flaps in three patients who were treated successfully by other techniques of reconstruction (Papineau and Ilizarov procedures). In the induced membrane and grafting procedure, bone healing was regularly obtained in a time that was independent of the length of reconstruction. In all cases the authors noted an aspect of radiological healing at 4 months. At the beginning of the authors'

experience, they performed additional grafts to reinforce the extremities of the reconstructed segment; but later the systematic petaling of the extremities permitted a primitive healing. At the lower limb, full weight bearing without protection was acquired in the mean time of 8.5 months (range: 6–17 months). Infection healed in all patients involved and that was probably in relation with the very radical initial debridement. In the series, the authors noted four stress fractures (2 early and 2 late) that healed by simple immobilization.

PROSPECTIVE CLINICAL STUDY

At the beginning of 2000, the authors thought that it could be interesting to associate local injection of recombinant human BMP-7 (Osigraft, Strycker, Biotech) with the bone autograft to enhance a quick formation of cortical bone.

From 2000 to 2004, 11 subjects had the two stages procedure for reconstruction of a wide diaphyseal defect. At the second stage, the morcellized cancellous bone autograft was mixed with a dose of 3.5 mg of eptotermin alpha and

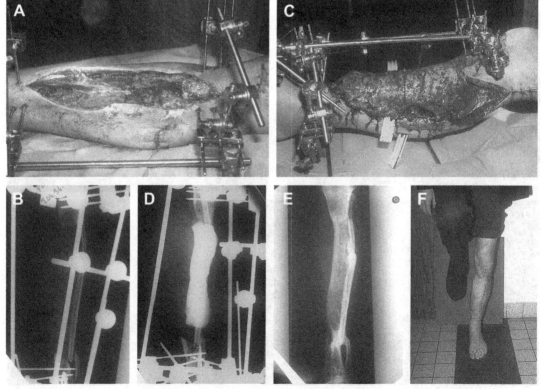

Fig. 3. Posttraumatic compound defect of the leg in a professional licensed pilot. (*A*) Initial aspect. (*B*) The segmental defect was 22 cm in length. (*C*) Soft-tissue envelope repair by a free flap. (*D*) The cement spacer under the flap. (*E*) Aspect of the reconstruction 2 years later; note the densification of the medial part of the graft according to Wolf's law. (*F*) Clinical aspect; this young man has succeeded in retrieving his license.

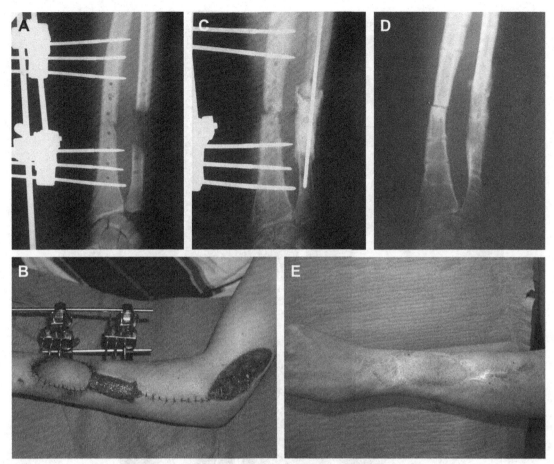

Fig. 4. Infected fracture of the forearm. (*A*) A segment of ulna was resected. (*B*) The soft-tissue defect was repaired by a custom made flap, the pedicle of which being supplied by the proximal cutaneous branch of the posterior interosseous artery. (*C*) The cement spacer under the flap. (*D, E*) Reconstruction healing and clinical aspect.

the preparation was left to the convenience of each surgeon. The series included 9 men and 2 women aged from 22 to 52 years (average 31). All the etiologies were posttraumatic septic nonunions. The segments involved were the tibia (9 cases), the femur (1 case), and the humerus (1 case). Bone defect ranged from 5 to 18 cm (average 10.5 cm). In eight cases the defect was segmental. Six subjects needed a soft-tissue repair by flaps (three latissimus dorsi free flaps; four muscle pedicled flaps). One subject had two pedicled flaps at the leg. Follow-up was more than 24 months for all subjects.

All flaps survived and no recurrence of infection occurred. Bone healing, implying a full weight bearing without protection for the lower segments, was obtained in the mean time of 11.5 months (6 to 18 months) for 10 subjects. One subject was amputated below the knee in a long-term evolution and a failure of consolidation. The most surprising was that three subjects developed a progressive deformity of the reconstructed tibial segment

a few months after what was considered the consolidation. Despite additional healing procedures, including prolonged immobilization by cast or external fixator, or intertibiofibular graft, a partial recurrence of the deformity occurred in two cases (**Fig. 5**).

Another peculiar event was the evolution of the radiological aspect of the bone graft in all subjects. The authors noted a quick densification at 2 months, then areas of clearness appeared in the reconstructed bone, which evoked partial and localized zones of resorption. The authors' conclusion was that the results of this series were not improved compared with their previous experience and that association with growth factors induced unexpected effects.

DISCUSSION
The Use of Additional Growth Factors

Recombinant human BMP-7 and recombinant human BMP-2 have been proved efficacious in

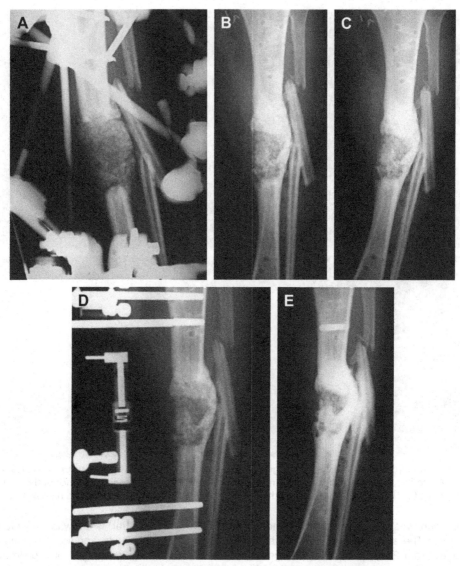

Fig. 5. Septic nonunion of the leg in a 20-year-old man. (*A*) Radiologic aspect after the bone graft associated with BMP-7. (*B*) The consolidation was considered as acquired at 8 months despite the inhomogeneous aspect of the reconstructed bone. (*C*) A varus deformity appeared progressively. (*D*) Reduction and stabilization by an external device which was maintained for 3 months. (*E*) Partial recurrence of the deformity after removing the external fixator.

improving accelerating bone healing in orthotopic animal models.[12] The BMP target is the perivascular connective tissue cells in the host bone bed. Clinical studies have also shown the possibility to repair segmental defects of the tibia by cancellous bone graft augmented with human morphogenetic protein[13] and to augment new-bone development.[14–16]

BMP-7 has been shown equivalent to autogenous iliac crest bone graft in a randomized prospective study of tibial fracture nonunions.[17] The efficacy of BMP-2 for treatment of open tibial fractures has been shown in a prospective,

randomized, controlled single-blind study[18] in accelerating bone healing and in reducing the need for secondary interventions. However, results of the authors' prospective study with BMP-7 are not encouraging.

Several reasons can be advanced to explain the absence of expected improvement with the addition of BMP-7; although several authors[18,19] claim that the bone morphogenetic protein implants have dose-dependent osteoinductive effect, the authors cannot infer that the delay of bone healing is caused by an insufficient dose of BMP. Other factors should be considered as the repartition of the BMP device inside the graft, the effect of post-operative aspiration drainage, and the lack of rigidity of the stabilization afforded by an external fixator. The presence of the membrane avoids the dispersion of the BMP device in the soft tissue and concentrates the substance inside the bone graft. Therefore, one can suppose some opposite action on osteoblast differentiation between TGF Beta 1 and BMP-7; although opposite effects have only been shown between TGF Beta 1 and BMP-2.[20]

On the other hand, even if BMP-7 is known to stimulate proliferation and differentiation of human bone cells in vitro, a high dose of BMP-7 inhibits the ALP (alkaline phosphatase) activity in the presence of vitamin D.[21] It can be supposed that the containment system of the membrane results in too high of a concentration of the BMP device.

Finally, according to the authors' clinical experience, they cannot determine the effect of the BMP-7 device on the healing of a bone autograft placed inside a membrane. The rather disappointing results of their clinical experience have incited them to delay the procedure using the BMP-7, while waiting to determine the conditions in using growth factors.

The Concept of Induced Membrane

The concept of induced membrane opens new perspectives. According to the results of the authors' first series and the fundamental studies, it can be asserted that induced membrane acts as a biological chamber. This assertion has recently been confirmed by independent experimental work.[22]

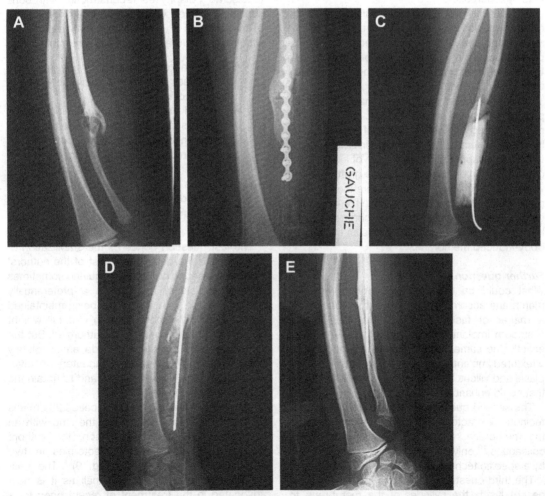

Fig. 6. Congenital pseudarthrosis of the ulna (*A*) Initial aspect. (*B*) Failure of a conventional treatment associating minimal resection, bone grafting and plating. (*C*) Radical excision sparing the distal growth plate and insertion of a cement spacer; stabilization by a wire. (*D*) Second stage; bone grafting after removing the spacer. (*E*) Radiologic aspect 3 years later; the ulnar growth plate remains open. (*Courtesy of* M.C. Romana, MD, Trousseau Hospital, Paris.)

The membrane prevents resorption of the cancellous bone while it is known that a large amount of cancellous bone placed in a richly vascularized muscular environment is partially or totally resorbed.[1,2,12] The membrane promotes the vascularization and the corticalization of the cancellous bone, even in bad vascularized bed like irradiated tissue or in very specific bone disease like congenital pseudarthrosis (**Fig. 6**). And finally, it is considered an in situ delivery system for growth and osteoinductive factors. The best period to perform the graft is 1 month after the set of the cement spacer.[9]

The induced membrane is quite different from the polylactide membranes. The latter can be used in association with a resorbable sponge[5] or cancellous bone graft.[6,7] Bone graft isolated from the soft tissue by a nonperforated membrane leads to necrosis.[7]

The conclusion of several studies is that the optimum device is a perforated, thin, and microporous membrane, and in large defects, the use of cancellous bone autograft in conjunction with fenestrated membrane produced the most consistent bone regenerate.[6,23]

However, these membranes have not been proven to secrete growth factors. Their mechanism is based on the exclusion of fibrous tissue inside the defects. Bone formation in small defects is probably supported by migration of local osteogenic cells. When cancellous bone graft is added within the lumen, small perforation of the membrane will allow the revascularization of the graft. Finally, the polylactide membranes do not have the same biological properties as the foreign body-induced membrane.

Further questions

What could be the most appropriate induced membrane according the type of the spacer? As a matter of fact, the membrane induced by a smooth implant like the PMMA cement is not exactly the same as the membrane induced by a textured implant. In the latter, synovial like metaplasia and villous hyperplasia are most developed that could enhance bone healing.

The second question is to search for other osteoinductive factors that could be secreted by the membrane. In the study of Pelissier and colleagues,[10] only the BMP-2 has been detected by a specific technique.

The third question is to determine what should be put inside the cylinder of the membrane to obtain the best reconstruction (ie, the quickest and the strongest one) from a mechanical point of view. Morcellized, fresh, cancellous bone autograft is probably the gold standard when

harvested from the iliac crests. In the authors' experience[4] the bone graft harvested from the four iliac crests allows reconstruction of a diaphyseal tibial defect up to 15 to 20 cm. No morbidity was noted at the donor site because the authors harvested the cancellous bone by appropriate skin incisions without raising any cortical block. In some cases, to preserve iliac crests, the authors added bone substitute with a ratio of 1:3; the authors did not observe a difference on rate of complication or time of healing with the reconstruction performed with cancellous bone alone (**Fig. 7**). Therefore, two important questions are: (1) which ratio of bone substitute is acceptable without compromising bone healing and mechanical strength, and (2) which is the most appropriate bone substitute? In other words, is the osteoinductivity of the membrane sufficient to assume a diaphyseal reconstruction with bone substitute alone? Other possibilities are worthy of interest and should be tested in association with the procedure of the induced membrane.

- Demineralized bone matrix has important properties combining osteoconductivity and osteoinductivity.[24]
- Intramedullary canal bone reamings (ICBR) can be used as a source of viable bone graft in relation to their osteoblastic potential and living bone cells similar to bone cells from the iliac crest.[25,26] The authors have recently started a prospective series of reconstruction associating induced membrane and ICBR from the femur (**Fig. 8**).

The last question concerns the stabilization of the limb and the defect. As most of the authors' cases were septic nonunions requiring sometimes iterative excisions, they chose a preferentially external fixator, with the device being maintained until the definitive bone healing and full weight bearing, without protection, is authorized. But the external fixator does not provide an absolutely rigid fixation, which seems mandatory to favor the action of the growth factors and to obtain the fusion of the bone graft.

Moreover, when the defect exceeds 20 cm it is difficult to maintain the axis of the limb with an external device. For that reason, the authors were obliged to perform osteotomies in two patients of the first series (**Fig. 9**).[4] The best solution is probably a locked nail as it is now advocated in the treatment of recent open fractures. But the nail raised other problems as the difficulty to remove the cement and the reduction of the space devoted to the massive reconstruction.

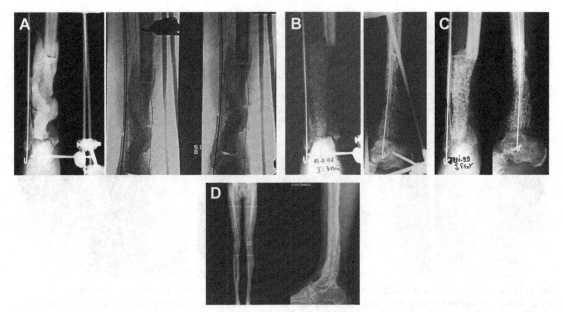

Fig. 7. Open fracture of the leg, stage IIIA Gustilo's classification. (*A*) Immediate huge bone defect—the fibula fracture was stabilized by a wire while the tibial defect was filled up with a cement spacer. (*B*) The postoperative course was uneventful, so that a huge graft was done 2 months later, consisting of fresh cancellous autograft and cancellous allograft with ratio of 50:50. Aspect of the recontruction at 3 months. (*C*) Aspect of the reconstruction at 10 months. External fixator was removed and free weight bearing was allowed. (*D*) Final result 6 years later.

SUMMARY

The authors think that the concept of membrane is well established as a bone reconstruction promotion by preventing the bone-graft resorption and by playing an important role in revascularization and consolidation. However, many problems remain to be solved relative to the stabilization, the type of material for reconstruction, the use of recombinant human growth factors, and the addition of stem cells.

Finally, this concept of membrane as a biological chamber could probably be extended to other tissular reconstruction as nerve grafting. This perspective fits in strangely with the poetic and philosophical vision of the organization of life of

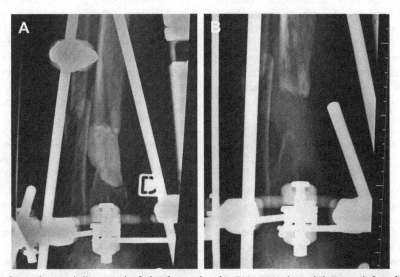

Fig. 8. Grafting from the medullar canal of the femur by the RIA procedure. (*A*) Bone defect filled up by the cement spacer. (*B*) At 3 months the graft seems well integrated. Partial weight bearing was allowed with protection of the external fixator.

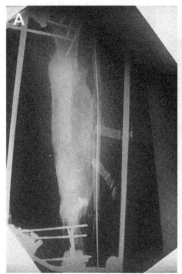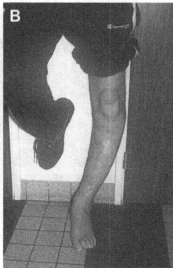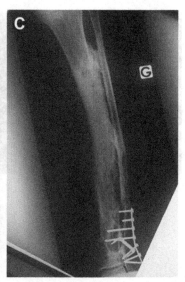

Fig. 9. Complication of a huge healed reconstruction of the tibia. (*A*) Initial bone defect was 24 cm length. (*B*) The varus deformity existed before the bone reconstruction and was caused by the difficulty to maintain the limb axis by an external fixator. Although the healing was acquired, the deformity was not acceptable from a mechanical point of view. (*C*) The correction of the deformity was obtained by a supramalleolar osteotomy.

Goethe who wrote in his book, *The Metamorphosis of Plants*: "A very important principle of the organization is that vital activity requires an envelope, which protects from the external elements. This envelope may be bark, skin, or shell, all that is living should be wrapped up."

REFERENCES

1. Hertel L, Gerber A, Schlegel U, et al. Cancellous bone graft for skeletal reconstruction muscular versus periosteal bed. Preliminary results. Injury 1994;25(Suppl 1):59–70.
2. Weiland AJ, Phillips TW, Randolph MA. Bone graft: a radiological, histological and biomechanical model comparing auto grafts, allografts and free vascularized bone grafts. Plast Reconstr Surg 1984;74:368–79.
3. Romana MC, Masquelet AC. Vascularized periosteum associated with cancellous bone graft: an experimental study. Plast Reconstr Surg 1990;85:587–92.
4. Masquelet AC, Fitoussi F, Bégué T, et al. Re construction des os longs par membrane induite et autogreffe spongieuse. Ann Chir Plast Esthet 2000;45:346–53 [in French].
5. Masquelet AC. Muscle reconstruction in reconstructive surgery: soft tissue repair and long bone reconstruction. Langenbecks Arch Surg 2003;388:344–6.
6. Ip WY. Polylactive membranes and sponges in the treatment of segmental defects in rabbit radii. Injury 2002;33(Suppl 2):66–70.
7. Gerber A, Gogolewski S. Reconstruction of large segmental defects in the sheep tibia using polylactide membranes. A clinical and radiographic report. Injury 2002;33(Suppl 2):43–57.
8. Gugal Z, Gogolewski S. Healing of critical size segmental bone defects in the sheep librae using bio resorbable polylactide membranes. Injury 2002;33(Suppl 2):71–6.
9. Klaue K, Anton C, Knothe U, et al. Biological implementation of "in situ" induced autologous foreign body membranes in consolidation of massive cancellous bone grafts. J Bone Joint Surg 1993;79B(Suppl II):236.
10. Pelissier P, Masquelet AC, Bareille R, et al. induced membranes secrete growth factors including vascular and osteoinductive factors and could stimulate bone regeneration. J Orthop Res 2004;22(1):73–9.
11. Pelissier P, Martin D, Baudet J, et al. Behavior of cancellous bone graft placed in induced membranes. Br J Plast Surg 2002;55:598–600.
12. Cook SD, Wolfe MW, Salked SL, et al. Effect of recombinant human osteogenic Protein-1 on healing of segmental defects in non-human primates. J Bone Joint Surg 1995;77A:734–50.
13. Johnson EE, Urist MR, Finerman GA. Repair of segmental defects of the tibia with cancellous bone grafts augmented with human bone morphogenetic protein. A preliminary report. Clin Orthop 1988;236:249–57.
14. Johnson EE, Urist AR, Finerman GA. Resistant non unions and partial or complete segmental defects of long bones. Treatment with implants of a composite of human bone morphogenetic protein

(BMP) and autolyzed, antigen-extract, allogenetic (AAA) bone. Clin Orthop 1992;277:229–37.

15. Cook SD, Barrack RL, Shimmin A, et al. The use of osteogenetic Protein-1 in reconstructive surgery of the hip. J Arthroplasty 2001;16(Suppl 1):88–94.

16. Cook SD, Barrack RL, Santman M, et al. Strut allograft healing to the femur with recombinant human osteogenic Protein-1. Clin Orthop 2000; 381:47–57.

17. Friedlander GE, Perry CR, Cole JD, et al. Osteogenic Protein-1 (bone morphogenetic Protein-7) in the treatment of tibial non unions. J Bone Joint Surg Am 2001;83(Suppl 1):151–8.

18. Salkeld SL, Patron LP, Barrack RL, et al. The effect of osteogenic Protein-1 on the healing of segmental bone defects treated with autograft or allograft bone. J Bone Joint Surg Am 2001;83:803–16.

19. BESTT Group, Govender S, Csimma C, et al. Recombinant human bone morphogenetic Protein-2 for treatment of open tibial fractures. J Bone Joint Surg Am 2002;84:2123–34.

20. Spinella-Jaegle S, Roman S, Faucheu C, et al. Opposite effects of bone morphogenetic protein 2 and transforming growth factor beta 1 on osteoblast differentiation. Bone 1998;29:323–30.

21. Knutsen R, Wergedal JE, Sampath TK, et al. Osteogenic Protein-1 stimulates proliferation and differentiation of human bone cells in vitro. Biochem Biophys Res Commun 1993;194: 1352–8.

22. Viateau V, Guillemin G, Calando Y, et al. Induction of a barrier membrane to facilitate reconstruction of massive segmental diaphyseal defect: an ovine model. Vet Surg 2006;35:445–52.

23. Meinig RP. Polylactide membranes in the treatment of segmental diaphyseal defects: animal model experiments in the rabbit radius, sheep tibia, Yucatan minipig radius, and goat tibia. Injury 2002; 33(Suppl 2):58–65.

24. Perterson B, Whang PJ, Iglesias R, et al. Osteo inductivity of commercially available demineralized bone matrix. J Bone Joint Surg Am 2004;86: 2243–50.

25. Tydings JD, Martino LJ, Kircher M, et al. The osteoinductive potential of intra medullary canal bone reamings. Curr Surg 1986;43:121–4.

26. Frolcke JP, Nulend JK, Semeins CM, et al. Viable osteoblastic potential of cortical reamings from intramedullary reaming. J Orthop Res 2004;22(6): 1271–5.

Clinical Use of Resorbable Polymeric Membranes in the Treatment of Bone Defects

Richard P. Meinig, MD

KEYWORDS

- Bone defect management
- Resorbable polymer membranes • Polylactide
- Guided • Bone regeneration

Large segmental defects remain a challenging clinical problem. Bone defects have many relevant clinical etiologies, such as high energy trauma, periprosthetic osteolysis, tumor resection, or osteomyelitis debridement. The goal of segmental bone defect reconstruction is to restore functional skeletal continuity and maintain soft-tissue function in a timely, well tolerated, and cost-effective manner. No single current technique is reliably successful in the reconstruction of large bone defects. Current strategies for the management of segmental bone defects include autogenous bone grafting, vascularized bone transfer, segmental allograft, demineralized bone matrix grafting, recombinant bone morphogenetic protein grafting, and numerous variants of distraction osteogenesis and bone transport.

Enhancing the local biologic environment to promote bone regeneration has long been recognized as efficacious. In the 1950s and 1960s investigations evaluated the use of nondegradable membranes to promote the healing of cortical defects.[1–3] The bone growth qualities of bulk porous materials, such as Teflon (polytetrafluoroethylene) and polyurethane sponges, was also studied during this time period.[4,5] The concept of membranes to enhance spontaneous bone regeneration emerged in the 1970s and 1980s in periodontal and craniomaxillofacial research.[6,7]

Periodontal bone loss has been clinically managed by the use of membranes to allow for the spontaneous regeneration of the periodontal ligament and tooth socket bone in a process that is described as guided tissue regeneration.[8] In addition, there were research efforts at promoting tissue regeneration, such as neural stints and vascular prostheses.[9,10]

The theoretical basis for using membranes to span segmental defects was, therefore, well established by the late 1980s. Initial animal studies confirmed the potential efficacy of membranes in critical-sized diaphyseal defects.[11] These membranes were fabricated with polylactide, which is a material with a long-established clinical history in orthopedic surgery as resorbable sutures. Microporous membranes were used as tubular stints that spanned diaphyseal defects of the rabbit radius. Membranes applied across a 1-cm segmental defect spontaneously healed with intralumenal woven bone and appositional bone formation along the outer membrane surface. Untreated defects failed to reconstitute and the defect filled with fibrous tissue and surrounding muscle (**Figs. 1** and **2**). The basic mechanisms for enhanced bone healing with membranes was demonstrated in the rabbit model as[1]: exclusion of nonosseous tissues,[2] maintenance of an osteogenic medullary canal, and[3]

Funding Support: The author currently receives no funding.

Department of Orthopedics, Front Range Orthopedic Association Memorial Hospital, 175 South Union, Suite 100, Colorado Springs, CO 80910, USA

E-mail address: rmeinig@comcast.net

Orthop Clin N Am 41 (2010) 39–47

doi:10.1016/j.ocl.2009.07.012

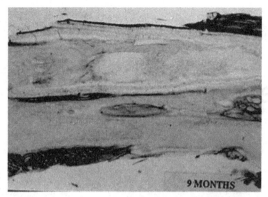

Fig.1. 1cm defect of rabbit radius treated with polylactide membrane. Cortical bone has formed along the membrane surface in continuity with the defect ends.

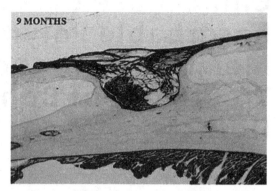

Fig. 2. 1cm defect of the rabbit radius untreated. Defect has filled with muscle and fibrous tissue. The defect ends have formed cortical caps.

the provision of a spatial scaffold for periosteal regeneration and revascularization.[12] Subsequent studies on larger defects of 2.5 to 7 cm in Yucatan minipig, goat, and sheep long bones showed that there was inconsistent spontaneous bone regeneration and that augmentation with autogenous bone graft was efficacious. In larger bone defects, revascularization from the surrounding soft tissues is a critical factor for defect healing with membranes. In addition, variables, such as membrane chemistry, resorption rates, membrane porosity, membrane thickness, and structure become increasingly important in larger defects. Numerous animal studies were performed to investigate these different membrane variables

and the supplemental modes of defect stabilization, such as external fixation, locked nails, and locked plates.[13–16] One of the most efficacious configurations studied was the use of two microporous (50–70 micrometer), poly (L/DL-lactide) meshed membranes (800–900 micrometer) to form a tube within a tube bridging a stabilized diaphyseal defect. The resultant space between the membranes, when grafted with autogenous bone graft, uniformly reconstituted a neocortex. The double membrane technique reduces the amount of autogenous bone needed to form a new cortical construct. In addition, bone formation was most extensive in the areas of the defect where there was an abundant muscle soft-tissue

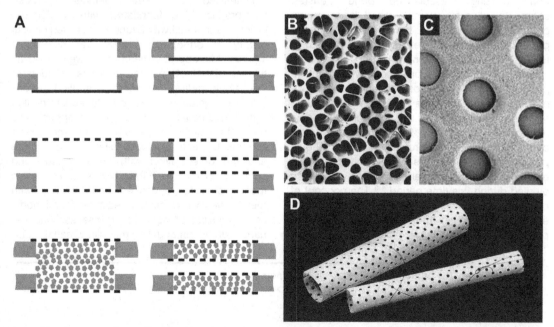

Fig. 3. Membrane configurations (A–D).

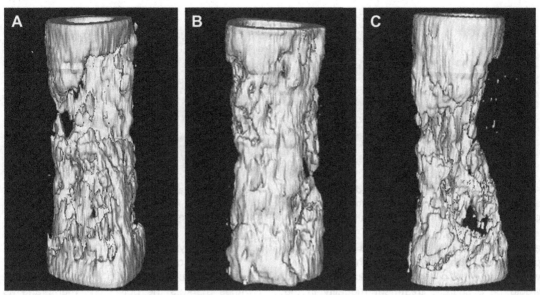

Fig. 4. CT reconstruction of bone regenerate (A–C).

envelope. The meshed membranes were efficacious in excluding soft-tissue invasion while allowing for vascular ingrowth. In addition, the mesh construct reduces the amount of polymer material to be resorbed.[17] Zibi fig. of membranes from Gugala and colleagues (**Figs. 3 and 4**).[18]

One of the primary clinical advantages of the polylactide membrane is its bioresorption. Because it is bioresorbable and biocompatible, there is no need for additional surgical explantation. The membrane is radiolucent to permit conventional radiographic, CT, and MRI of the bone regeneration. In addition, the bioresorption eliminates any potential effects of stress shielding. The animal studies confirmed that the degradation of polylactide membranes into local lactic acid, and ultimately water and carbon dioxide, was well tolerated by the host. Numerous histologic specimens among various animal species demonstrated early incorporation of the membrane by regenerate bone without an inflammatory response (**Fig. 5**). Membranes that were loaded with calcium carbonate ($CaCO_3$) demonstrated the feasibility of adding bone mineral substrate for additional osteoconductive and biologic activity (**Fig. 6**). Membranes could also be heat molded into various tubular structures or curved surfaces as needed to fit the clinical defect (**Fig. 7**). At the conclusion of the animal studies, membrane chemical composition, porosity, and gross structure, such as thickness and meshing, had been adequately studied for the fabrication of a membrane that was suitable for human implantation. In addition, membranes had been studied with and without bone graft, with plate stabilization, intramedullary (IM) nail stabilization,

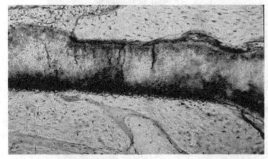

Fig. 5. High power magnification of membrane-bone interface. Bone has formed in apposition to membrane surfaces without inflammatory or fibrous cell reaction.

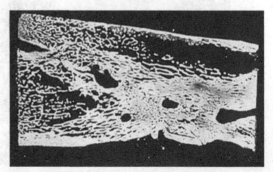

Fig. 6. Bone formed in a 3cm defect of the minipig radius treated with a polylactide membrane loaded with $CaCO_3$.

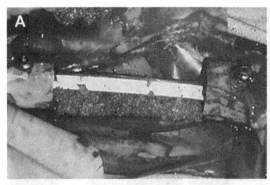
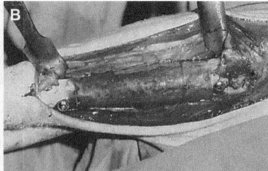

Fig. 7. (*A*). Sheep tibia defect stabilized with locked unreamed intramedullary (IM) nail with iliac crest autograft and microporous polylactide membrane. (*B*) Sheep defect with membrane formed as a tube and filled with iliac crest bone graft. Membrane form maintained by cerclage suture at margins.

and in situ for small defects. Thus, it appeared that polylactide mesh membranes, when combined with stable fixation and autogenous bone graft, would be a suitable treatment modality in the human clinical situation.

CLINICAL TECHNIQUE AND EXPERIENCE
Material

Presently, Synthes manufactures polylactide membranes for clinical implantation. For craniomaxillofacial applications, Synthes Synmesh has been available for treatment of bone defects and orbital wall blow-out fractures. For long bone applications, Synthes markets the polylactide membrane as "OrthoMesh Resorbable Graft Containment System" (Synthes US, Paoli, PA). The Synthes product is composed of 85:15 poly (L-lactide-co-glycolide) that has been formed into a membrane that is 0.5 mm thick and has been perforated with holes to form a mesh. The polymer degrades into lactic and glycolic acid and ultimately to

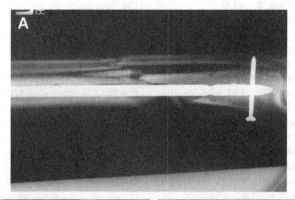

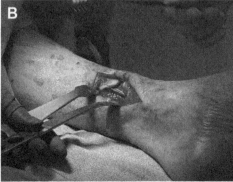
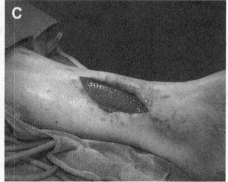

Fig. 8. (*A*) Near circumferential cortical defect at diaphyseal metaphyseal junction in Grade II open fracture at 8 weeks. (*B*) Surgical exposure of medial aspect of defect. (*C*) Polylactide membrane-mesh formed as a ¾ tube and filled with iliac crest bone graft harvested with acetabular reamer.

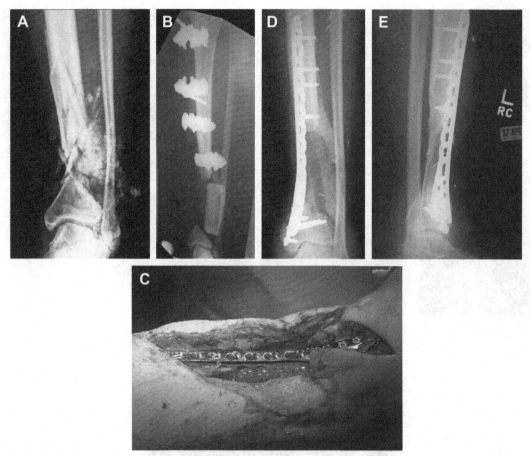

Fig. 9. (*A*) High-energy distal tibia fracture. (*B*) External fixation of distal tibia with placement of antibiotic-polymethyl methacrylate (PMMA) spacer and flap coverage. (*C*) Defect following antibiotic spacer removal, fixation with a spanning locked plate, RIA autogenous bone graft, and a double tube construct with polylactide mesh. (*D, E*) Anterior-posterior radiograph and lateral radiographs at 7 months postoperative showing reconstitution of bone defect.

carbon dioxide and water. The membrane mesh has an in vivo lifespan of approximately 12 months and maintains approximately 85% of its bending strength after 8 weeks. The mesh is sterilized and is available as a 50 × 50 mm or 100 mm × 100 mm sheet. The mesh can be cut to size intraoperatively with scissors. In addition, a sterile hot water bath tray is provided so that the membrane becomes pliable for in vivo molding and contouring for the clinical defect.

Autogenous Bone Graft

Harvesting adequate and viable bone graft is likely instrumental for success. The iliac crest has long been recognized as the gold standard for autogenous cancellous bone. The anterior or posterior iliac crest can be harvested in a conventional manner with curettes and osteotomes. A small hip arthroplasty acetabular reamer can be used to harvest bone graft from the anterior iliac crest.[19] This technique provides copious bone graft in a paste like slurry that handles well for filling defects.

More recently, the Reamer-Irrigator-Aspirator (RIA) has been used to harvest large amounts of autogenous bone graft. In this technique, a single pass reaming is performed of the femur or tibia with a suction irrigated reamer (Synthes USA, Paoli, PA). The reamer shavings are collected and typically yield 40 to 70 mL of highly osteogenic slurry that can be used for defect filling.[20]

The addition of demineralized bone matrix allograft materials or human recombinant bone morphogenetic proteins to the autogenous bone graft can also be performed. The optimum ratio and clinical indications and efficacy at this point have not been determined.

Implantation

Implantation of a membrane with autogenous bone graft offers the clinician an opportunity to

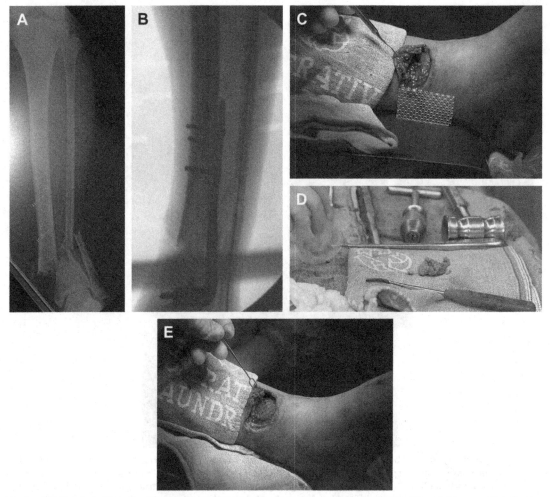

Fig. 10. (*A, B*) Injury film of open Grade IIIb fracture treated with initial external fixation. Intraoperative fluoroscopic view of locked plating and harvesting autogenous bone with RIA. (*C, D, E*) Implantation of polylactide mesh with RIA autograft.

treat bone loss as a single step procedure. The long bone defect or metaphyseal defect is stabilized per physician preference with restoration and maintenance of length, angular alignment, and rotation. Diaphyseal defects can be fixed with a double locked IM nail, locked plate, or external fixator construct. Similarly, metaphyseal defects can be stabilized with conventional implants. The defect is then exposed and debrided, if necessary, of interposed scar and fibrous tissue. Care is taken to minimize any surgical trauma to the soft tissue envelope of skin and surrounding muscle. After creating a suitable cavity for bone grafting the membrane is prepared. The membrane mesh is cut with sterile scissors to overlap the cortical ends by approximately 1 cm. The sterile water bath is heated to 70°C. The mesh is then immersed in the bath for approximately 15–20 seconds to allow the mesh to become pliable. The membrane can be rolled into a tubular shape or other shape to best approximate the defect. The defect is bridged or covered with the mesh. The ends of the mesh can be affixed with circumferential suture or tack sutures as needed. If a tube within a tube construct is being made, a second mesh tube is made by immersion into the heated water bath and the tube rolled to fit the medullary canal of both ends of the defect. Bone graft is then harvested either using the acetabular reamer technique to harvest iliac bone graft or the RIA technique to harvest bone graft from the femur or tibia. The bone graft is then immediately transferred to the defect, which is packed as a single cavity or as a neocortex between double meshes. The mesh is closed upon itself or used as cover over a cavitary defect. The tubular construct is sutured closed with a minimal number of resorbable

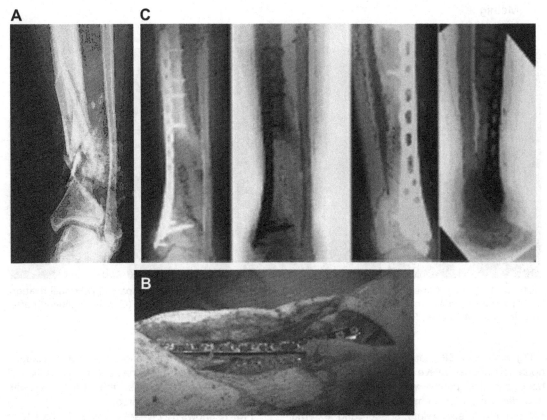

Fig. 11. (*A*) Injury films. (*B*) Conversion from temporary external fixation to plate, RIA bone graft, and membrane. (*C*) Healed defect.

sutures. The surgical incision is then closed over suction drainage, which is maintained for 24 to 48 hours. A soft dressing with a splint, if needed, is applied to hold the limb in neutral alignment. Conventional antibiotic prophylaxis for 24 hours is instituted. Patients can be mobilized with functional therapy and weight bearing as clinically indicated. In one known case, a vascularized muscle flap was applied over a membrane at 6 weeks without complication.

Clinical Examples

CC

Fig. 8 shows a 54-year-old male with grade IIIB open tibia fracture, initially treated with an unreamed nail. The patient had a defect of 3cm involving the anterior and medial aspect of the distal tibia at the diaphyseal and metaphyseal junction. Definitive treatment consisted of conversion to reamed retrograde nail with an autologous iliac bone graft, and tubular mesh bridging defect.

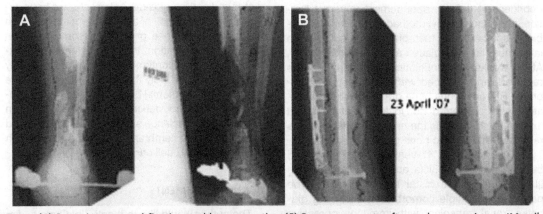

Fig. 12. (*A*) Spanning external fixation and bone resection (*B*) Bone regenerate after early conversion to IM nail, free flap coverage, RIA bone grafting and membrane implantation.

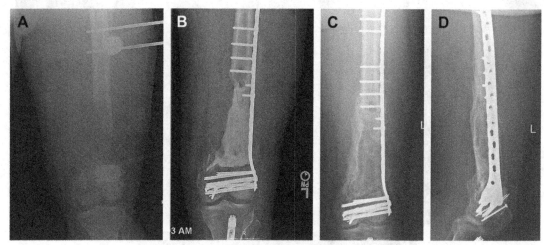

Fig. 13. (*A*) Diaphyseal bone loss of distal femur treated with initial debridement and spanning external fixation. (*B*) Conversion from external fixation to plate fixation with PMMA antibiotic spacer. (*C*) Bone regenerate after removal of PMMA spacer, RIA bone grafting and membrane implantation (*D*).

Fig. 9 shows a 38-year-old male with grade IIIB open tibia and extensive diaphyseal metaphyseal bone loss. The patient was initially treated with debridement and placement of antibiotic impregnated methylmethacrylate spacer and external fixation. Definitive treatment occurred at 6 weeks with a conversion to locked plate, RIA autograft, and double tube construct of polylactide mesh membranes to form a tube within a tube.

Fig. 10 shows a 40-year-old male with a Grade IIIB open distal tibia metaphyseal fracture. The patient was initially treated with spanning external fixation, converted to locked plate, RIA bone graft of ipsilateral tibia, and membrane cover of anterior medial bone defect. Skin loss with vascularized muscle coverage occurred at 6 weeks postmesh implantation.

Fig. 11 shows a 32-year-old male with a Grade IIIB fracture of the distal tibia and fibula. The patient was initially treated with irrigation and debridement (I & D), debridement, external fixation, and a polymethyl methacrylate (PMMA) antibiotic spacer for a metaphyseal defect. A free latissimus flap was placed at 2 weeks postinjury. At 10 weeks, the antibiotic PMMA spacer was removed, and replaced with a polylactide membrane; RIA antologus bone graft. The external fixator was converted to locked plate internal fixation. At 15 months the residual bone void was regrafted with an iliac bone graft.

Fig. 12 shows a 47-year-old male who had been in a motor vehicle accident with a Grade IIIA fracture of the distal tibia and fibula. The patient has multiple comorbidities including diabetes, renal transplant with immunosuppressive therapy, and smoking. Initial treatment consisted of I & D, and external fixation. The external fixation was converted to an IM nail and fibula fixation at 72 hours. At 10 weeks, the RIA graft, with a membrane, was implanted.

Fig. 13 shows a 27-year-old male who had been in a motorcycle accident with a Grade IIIa open fracture and bone loss. Initial treatment was debridement and spanning external fixation. The patient converted to plate fixation with a PMMA antibiotic spacer with subsequent RIA bone grafting and membrane implantation.

SUMMARY

Resorbable polymer membranes of the poly (lactide) chemical class are a promising technique for single-step reconstruction of large bone defects. Poly (lactides) have long been used in human cases where the material is harmlessly metabolized to lactic acid, and subsequently, water and carbon dioxide. Animal studies have established the efficacy of a meshed membrane with an autogenous bone graft when combined with stable internal fixation. Initial implantation in clinical cases has confirmed that a commercially available meshed poly (lactide) is effective in the treatment of segmental bone defects. Further clinical use will further define the technique.[18,20,21] In addition, basic science studies will further expand the potential for membrane fabrication as a growth factor, drug, and cell carrier.

ACKNOWLEDGMENTS

The author would like to thank Zibi Gugala, Jim Green, Thomas Higgins, Gary Rosenberg, and

Sylwester Gogolewski for basic science or clinical case material.

REFERENCES

1. Lindhome WJ. The sequence of events in osteogenesis as studied in polyethylene tubes. Ann N Y Acad Sci 1960;85:445–60.
2. Goldhaber P. Osteogenic induction across millipore filters in vivo. Science 1961;133:2065–7.
3. Ruedi TP, Basset CA. Repair and remodeling in millipore isolated defects in cortical bone. Acta Anat 1967;68:509–31.
4. Gilmer WS, Tooms RE, Salvatore JE. An experimental study of the influence of polyurethane sponges upon subsequent bone formation. Surg Gynecol Obstet 1961;114:143–8.
5. Friedenberg ZB, Simon WH. Bone Growth in teflon Sponge. Surg Gynecol Obstet 1963;116:588–92.
6. Magnusson I, Batich C, Collins B. New attachment formation following controlled tissue regeneration using biodegradable membranes. J Clin Periodontol 1988;59:1–5.
7. Dahlin C, Gottlow L, Karring T, et al. Healing of mandibular and maxillary bone defects using a membrane technique: an experimental study in monkeys. Scand J Plast Reconstr Surg Hand Surg 1990;24:13–9.
8. Eickholz P, Pretzle B, Holle R, et al. Long term results of guided tissue regeneration therapy with nonresorbable and bioabsorbable barrier: function after 10 years. J Periodontol 2006;77:88–94.
9. Mackinnon SM. New directions in peripheral nerve repair. Ann Plast Surg 1989;22:257–73.
10. Gogolewski S, Galletti G, Ussia G. Polyurethane vascular prosthesis in pigs. Colloid Polym Sci 1987;265:774–8.
11. Meinig RP, Rahn B, Perren SM, et al. Regeneration of diaphyseal bone defects using a resorbable poly(L-lactide) tissue separation membrane. Int J Artif Organs 1990;13:577.
12. Meinig RP, Rahn B, Perren SM, et al. Bone regeneration with resorbable polymeric membranes: treatment of diaphyseal bone defects in the rabbit radius with poly(L-lactide) membrane. J Orthop Trauma 1996;10:178–90.
13. Meinig RP, Buesing CM, Helm J, et al. Regeneration of diaphyseal bone defects using poly(L/DL-lactide) and poly(D-lactide) membranes in the Yucatan pig model. J Orthop Trauma 1997;11(8):551–8.
14. Pineda LM, Buesing CM, Meinig RP, et al. Bone regeneration with resorbable polymer membranes. III. Effect of poly (L-lactide) membrane pore size on the bone healing of large bone defects. J Biomed Mater Res 1996;31:385–94.
15. Gogolewski S, Manil-Varlet P, Pineda LM, et al. Bone regeneration with resorbable polymer membranes. IV. Does the chemical composition of the membrane affect the healing process. J Biomed Mater Res 2000;21:2513–20.
16. Gerber A, Gogolewski S. Reconstruction of large segmental defects in sheep tibia using polylactide membranes. A clinical and radiographic report. Injury 2002;33(2):43–57.
17. Gugala Z, Gogolewski S. Healing of critical-size segmental bone defects in the sheep tibiae using bioresorbable polylactide membranes. Injury 2002;33(2):71–6.
18. Gugala Z, Lindsay R, Gogolewsks S. New approaches in the treatment of critical-size segmental defects in long bones. Macromolecular Symposia 2007;253:147–61.
19. Dick W. Use of the acetabular reamer to harvest autogenic bone graft material: a simple method for producing bone paste. Arch Orthop Trauma Surg 1986;185:225–8.
20. Hammer TO, Wieling R, Green JM, et al. Effect of reimplanted particles from Intramedullary reaming on mechanical properties and callus formation. A laboratory study. J Bone Joint Surg 2007;89B:1534–8.
21. Ip WY, Gogolewski S. Clinical applications of resorbable polymers in guided bone regeneration. Macromolecular Symposia 2007;252:139–46.

Use of the Induced Membrane Technique for Bone Tissue Engineering Purposes: Animal Studies

Véronique Viateau, DMV, PhD[a],*, Morad Bensidhoum, PhD[b],
Geneviève Guillemin, PhD[b], Hervé Petite, PhD[b],
Didier Hannouche, DM, PhD[c], Fani Anagnostou, DM[b],
Philippe Pélissier, DM[d]

KEYWORDS
- Bone • Tissue engineering • Coraline scaffolds
- Bone graft • Critical-size bone defects

Clinical management of extensive segmental long-bone defects occurring after high-energy trauma or debridement for infected nonunion poses a substantial orthopedic challenge. Current solutions include the use of cancellous autografts when defects are 4 to 5 cm or smaller, whereas other procedures such as transfer of vascularized bone or intercalary bone transport methods are required to treat longer defects.[1–3]

Masquelet and colleagues[4,5] reported successful repair of wide diaphyseal defects (≤25 cm) with concurrent severe soft tissue loss in human patients using fresh autologous cancellous bone grafts in an original two-step surgical procedure. In the first step, a polymethylmethacrylate (PMMA) cement spacer was inserted into the defect inducing formation of an encapsulation membrane. After 8 weeks, the spacer was removed and the cavity filled with autologous cancellous graft harvested from the iliac crest. Bone union was usually achieved within 8.5 months, with patients recovering normal gait and motion. Interestingly, the procedure applied to all sorts of defects in contrast to the use of a massive allograft. Clinical trials in which the procedure has been performed have highlighted the advantages of using the induced membrane: (1) prevention of protrusion of adjacent soft tissues in the bone defect; (2) restraint of the graft in place; and, according to Masquelet,[4] (3) maintenance of graft volume over time through either protection of the graft against resorption or local production of osteoinductive substances.[6] Interestingly, animal studies have demonstrated that the membrane indeed has histologic characteristics and biologic properties that might facilitate bone healing.[7,8]

Large quantities of autograft and sometimes repeated surgery to achieve bone union are nevertheless needed for successful outcome with this procedure. The development of tissue-engineered bone constructs (TEBC) combining osteoconductive scaffolds with autologous mesenchymal stem cells (MSC), the availability of bone morphogenetic proteins, have opened new avenues for designing efficient bone substitutes. The possibility of placing either skeletal stem cells or bone

[a] Unité Pédagogique de Pathologie Chirurgicale, Ecole vétérinaire d'Alfort, 94700 Maisons-Alfort, France
[b] Laboratoire de Bioingénierie et Biomécanique Ostéo-articulaires (LB2OA), Université Paris Diderot, Paris 7, 10 Avenue de Verdun, 75010 Paris, France
[c] Service de Chirurgie Orthopédique, Hôpital Lariboisière, 75010 Paris, France
[d] Service de Chirurgie Plastique–Main, Centre F.X. Michelet, Groupe Hospitalier Pellegrin, 33076 Bordeaux, France
* Corresponding author.
E-mail address: vviateau@vet-alfort.fr (V. Viateau).

Orthop Clin N Am 41 (2010) 49–56
doi:10.1016/j.ocl.2009.07.010
0030-5898/09/$ – see front matter © 2010 Published by Elsevier Inc.

morphogenetic proteins (BMPs) onto scaffolds in the cavity delineated by the membrane is a very attractive prospect.

The purpose of this article was to review data from animal studies that have allowed better understanding of the structure and properties of the membrane as well as the preliminary and preclinical evaluations of new therapeutic strategies using the induced membrane procedure.

ANIMAL MODELS USING THE INDUCED MEMBRANE PROCEDURE

The structure and biologic properties of the induced membrane have been studied in small (rabbit) and large (sheep) animal species in which implantation of PMMA cylinders in either the dorsal paraspinal subcutaneous tissue (ectopic implantation sites) or segmental bone defects (orthotopic implantation sites) have induced the formation of a membrane. These animal models have been further used to assess the osteogenic potential of different TEBC.

Ectopic Models

Subcutaneous implantation of PMMA cylinders (four 10-mm-diameter, 5-mm-long cylinders in rabbits, eighteen 15-mm-diameter, 28-mm-long cylinders in sheep), have made possible the analysis of the structure and biologic characteristics of the induced membrane at different time points after cement implantation.[7,9]

Briefly, induced membranes were sampled at different time points postoperatively (2, 4, 6, and 8 weeks in rabbit experiments; 6 and 14 weeks in sheep experiments) and processed for histology and immunohistochemical analysis to assess structure and inflammatory reaction. Samples from membranes induced in sheep were immunostained to assess the presence of Col-1 and vascular endothelial growth factor (VEGF), as well as CD14 (for macrophages) and CBFA-1 (for osteoblast precursor cells) positive cells. Samples from membranes induced in rabbits were processed for protein extraction and dosage of growth factors (VEGF, transforming growth factor [TGF]-β1, BMP-2). Proliferation and differentiation of human bone marrow stromal cells grown into a culture medium containing protein extracts from either the induced membrane or subcutaneous tissue (controls) were also evaluated.

Orthotopic Models

Implantation of PMMA cylinders in either 25-mm-long metatarsal or 30-mm-long femoral segmental bone critical size bone defects (CSD) stabilized with a bone plate in sheep has made possible the validation of the procedure described by Masquelet and colleagues using morselized corticocancellous bone autograft in conditions similar to the one encountered in clinical situations (eg, replacement of a CSD in a load-bearing bone, in an animal with bone healing and remodeling characteristics close to humans').[6,8] Briefly, a mid-diaphyseal segmental bone resection was created and filled with a cement spacer for 4 or 6 weeks. At these time points, the cement was carefully removed through an incision made along the formed encapsulation membrane surrounding the cement, and the resultant cavities were either left empty or filled with a morselized autologous bone graft sampled from the iliac crest. Bone healing was obtained in both femoral and metatarsal defects within 4 to 6 months, respectively. Membrane induced at the metatarsal site was sampled and processed for histology and immunohistochemistry at time of cement removal and bone grafting, 6 weeks postoperatively, and at the time the animals were humanely killed 6 months later, making possible the characterization of its structure in a bone site.

CHARACTERISTICS AND BIOLOGIC PROPERTIES OF THE INDUCED MEMBRANE: DATA FROM ANIMAL EXPERIMENTS
Macroscopic Characteristics

Both subcutaneous and orthotopic implantation of PMMA cylinders in rabbit and sheep experiments induced the formation of a fibrous membrane. Implantation in ectopic and orthotopic sites in sheep have shown that at time of cement removal, 6 weeks after cement implantation, the membrane was 1 to 2 mm thick, not adherent to underlying cement thus allowing easy removal of the later and bled when incised. It was also mechanically competent in both locations and incised edges could be sutured without tension thus delineating a cavity in which either bone autograft or TEBC could be contained.[8,9]

As shown in sheep in which PMMA cylinders were implanted into segmental metatarsal bone defects, the encapsulation membrane prevented adjacent soft tissue protrusion in the defect. In these experiments, the membrane was indeed found adherent to the resected bone edges and did not collapse after cement removal, thus delineating a cavity corresponding to the volume of the retrieved cement spacer. This was an important outcome because it has been reported that the use of pliable and nonrigid membranes (ie, silicone sheeting) across a defect may result in nonunions because of collapse of the membrane and subsequent interposition of tissue in the defect.[10]

Interestingly, the membrane defined the shape of the regenerating bone as replacement bone retained the original size and contour along the defect throughout the study. The induced membrane indeed constrained the autograft, which was a critical issue, as in human patients, a major problem encountered with use of morselized graft for segmental bone losses greater than 4 cm long is constraint of bone chips to the site and prevention of soft tissue protrusion into the defect.[5]

At last, use of an enclosed space to constrain autologous bone chips within the defect prevented ectopic bone formation. This is of particular relevance in tissue engineering strategies where maintenance of biologic agents within defect areas is critical.

Histologic and Immunohistochemical Characteristics

Histologic and immunohistochemical analysis of membrane specimens sampled 6 weeks after subcutaneous or orthotopical implantation of PMMA cylinders in both rabbit and sheep models have shown that the induced membrane was made of a collagenous matrix in which numerous elongated fibroblasticlike cells were found embedded (**Fig. 1**). Collagen fibers were orientated parallel to the PMMA surface.

The membrane was highly vascularized in both ectopic and orthotopic sites (**Fig. 2**). A mild inflammatory reaction with the presence of multinucleated giant cells was observed within induced membranes in subcutaneous and bone sites. Subcutaneous implantation of PMMA cylinders in rabbits showed that it decreased from 2 to 8 weeks postoperatively.[7] These observations were further confirmed in sheep in which inflammatory cells were identified within encapsulation membranes in subcutaneous membranes sampled at time of cement removal (6 weeks) and constructs explantation (14 weeks postoperatively).[9] Immunoreactivity for CD14 was not observed in 6-month membrane explants from sheep having undergone bone grafting using the induced membrane procedure in metatarsal location suggesting that at that time point, the inflammatory reaction had ceased.[8]

The mild inflammatory reaction in the membranes induced experimentally is an interesting observation in tissue engineering. It differs from the histologic response observed when silicone spacers were used as an interposition material for reconstruction of traumatic bone loss in humans.[11] The later indeed included T cell and macrophage reactions, with foreign-body giant cells embedded in a vascularized pseudosynovium. Silicone debris was frequently observed under polarized light in the connective tissue and within giant multinucleated cells.[12,13] A similar foreign-body reaction has been reported after use of liquid PMMA (instead of the dough PMMA cement we used) implanted around cemented hip implants,[14] and for kyphoplasty.[15]

Although foreign body reaction within PMMA-induced membrane remained mild in animal experiments, further investigation is yet needed to test the hypothesis that the membrane can protect bone graft or resorbable osteoconductive

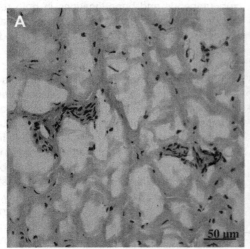
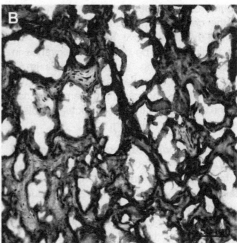

Fig. 1. Immunohistochemical staining of the encapsulation membrane sampled at time of cement explantation from a sheep metatarsal defect (*A*). Type I collagen staining shows that the membrane is mainly composed of an alveolar organization of parallel bands of collagen fibers (*B*).

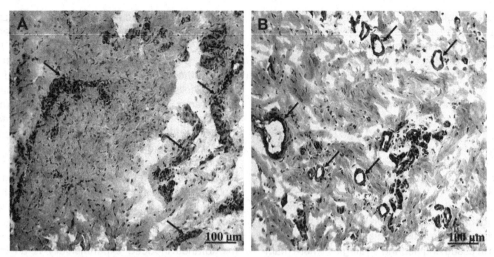

Fig. 2. Immunohistochemical staining of the encapsulation membrane sampled at time of cement explantation from a sheep metatarsal defect. *Lycopersicon esculentum* lectin labeling of vessels in longitudinal (*A*) and transverse (*B*) sections demonstrating the perpendicular orientation of the membrane vascularization (*arrows*).

materials from premature resorption as some authors have suggested.[6]

Biologic Properties

Animal experiments have pointed out biologic characteristics that may be of clinical interest for tissue-engineering purposes.

Secretion of angiogenic factors

Protein extraction from membranes induced after subcutaneous PMMA implantation in rabbits has shown a higher concentration of VEGF compared with control subcutaneous samples. Furthermore, it was found that membranes induced in subcutaneous and bone sites were highly vascularized in both rabbit and sheep. Interestingly, vessels were found oriented perpendicular to the long axis of the cement implanted in the metatarsal site, toward the bone defect (**Fig. 2**).

These findings may be of clinical relevance in bone tissue engineering, as angiogenesis is an essential step in osteogenesis. However, the hypothesis that the encapsulation membrane has a substantial role in graft or constructs vascularization remains to be validated.

Osteoinductive and/or osteogenic properties

Osteoinductive or osteogenic properties have been attributed to the induced membrane.

Protein extraction from membranes induced after subcutaneous PMMA implantation in rabbits have shown that they contained a higher concentration of TGF-β1 at different time points (2, 4, 6, and 8 weeks postoperatively) and of BMP-2 (4 and 6 weeks postoperatively) compared with control subcutaneous samples. It has further

been shown that protein extraction from these membranes promoted human MSC proliferation and differentiation into bone-forming cells.[7] BMP-2 production was found a maximum of 4 weeks postoperatively, suggesting that there might be an optimal time for bone grafting.

In one experiment in sheep in which cement spacers were implanted in segmental metatarsal defects, fibroblastlike cells positive for CBFA1, a critical transcription factor for osteoblast differentiation, were identified throughout the encapsulation membranes collected from two sheep at time of PMMA removal.[8] These cells were not found in membranes induced subcutaneously. Yet, neither woven nor mature bone was found in the core of the encapsulation membranes in subcutaneous and bone locations in both rabbit and sheep experiments.[7,9] Some bone formation did occur occasionally from the bone defect edges on the internal side of, but not within, the membranes.

Interestingly, sheep femoral bone defects left empty after removal of the cement spacer 4 weeks postoperatively, showed higher bone formation, 4 months postoperatively, when the induced membrane was preserved compared with defects in which the membrane had been resected at time of cement removal. Similar trends have been observed in metatarsal defects. Yet, in the latter, different observation time periods between defects with (6 months) and without (4 months) preservation of the induced membrane have prevented objective comparisons. In all cases, bone formation though remained limited and confined to the internal aspect of the membrane, in the close vicinity of resected cortices suggesting that the membrane per se had limited bone-regeneration capacity. Further investigation is therefore needed to test the hypothesis that the encapsulation membrane does have a substantial osteogenic role.

Maintenance of graft volume

As observed in clinical studies in humans, morselized bone autografts used to fill the cavity delineated by the membrane in femoral and metatarsal segmental defects in sheep retained their original shape and size throughout the studies (4 and 6 months, respectively), grossly matching the ones of the resected bone (**Fig. 3**).[6,8]

Whether maintenance of graft volume in the cavity delineated by the induced membrane results from (1) higher new bone formation; (2) lesser graft resorption; (3) prevention of adjacent tissue protrusion in the defect; or (4) prevention of graft migration within soft tissues surrounding the bone defect, remains to be established. Interestingly, whereas substantial graft resorption occurred when the membrane was removed before grafting in femoral defects in sheep, this was not observed in metatarsal defects in which similar bone replacement volumes were obtained when the induced membrane was resected before grafting. The metatarsal defect is well delineated by strong extensor and flexor tendons on its dorsal and plantar aspects, respectively, and by skin on its lateral and medial aspects; protrusion of these tissues in the defect is unlikely and the graft is naturally constrained in such a well-delineated cavity. In contrast, the femoral defect is surrounded by heavy muscles, which makes it difficult to delineate a cavity in which the graft remains. Thus, preservation of the induced membrane may be a more critical issue in situations in which creation of a well-delineated closed space and prevention of adjacent tissue protrusion is difficult to obtain.

NEW PERSPECTIVES IN BONE TISSUE ENGINEERING USING THE INDUCED MEMBRANE TECHNOLOGY

The histologic characteristics and the biologic properties of the induced membrane provide an attractive environment for the evaluation of TEBC. Advances in bone tissue repair have indeed highlighted the conditions that must be fulfilled for successful segmental bone loss replacement to occur: (1) prevention of soft tissue protrusion in the defect; (2) scaffold for osteoconduction; (3) maintenance of adequate vascularization in the defect; and (4) creation of a closed space in which osteogenic cells and substances are retained, thus promoting new bone deposition.[16,17] Constructs in a granular form (allowing replacement of a wide variety of defects in terms of volume and shape) and in clinically relevant volumes (to simulate clinical situations) have been evaluated either

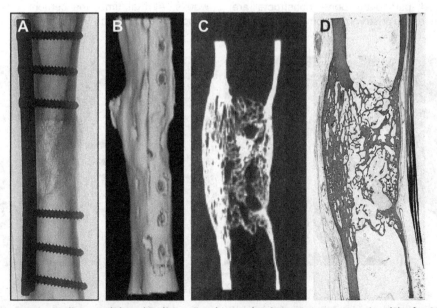

Fig. 3. Representative radiogram (*A*) and 3-dimensional tomodensitometry reconstruction (*B*) of a 25-mm-long metatarsal critical size defect of a sheep implanted with fragmented autologous bone, 6 months after cement removal. Microradiography (frame *C*), and histology (*D*) of a representative 2-dimensional section were performed at this time point. The stain used for the histology was van Gieson picro-fushine.

ectopically in preliminary trials (to assess their osteogenic potential) or orthotopically in preclinical trials in rabbit and sheep experiments.

Use of the Induced Membrane Technique to Evaluate Osteogenic Potential of Bone Tissue Engineered Constructs

Hybrid constructs combining porous scaffolds and bone morphogenetic protein

The biologic effect of induced membranes on cylindrical-shaped hydroxyapatite/tricalcium phosphate (HA-TCP) implants loaded with rhOP-1 was studied by Pélissier and colleagues[18] in a rabbit subcutaneous model. Briefly, 60% HA-40% TCP implants, either plain or loaded with rhOP-1, were implanted in the back of rabbits, either in a subcutaneous tunnel or within a subcutaneous PMMA-induced membrane. Implants were excised and analyzed for bone formation, 4 and 16 weeks postoperatively. None of the plain implants showed any evidence of bone formation suggesting that the induced membrane per se did not have any osteogenic property. Interestingly, bone ingrowth within implants loaded with BMP-7 was significantly higher when implants were inserted into induced membranes compared with implants inserted in subcutaneous tunnels, suggesting that the membrane may affect osteogenesis in the presence of BMP-7.

Hybrid constructs combining coralline scaffolds and autologous mesenchymal stem cells

Standardized particulate bone constructs are simpler to use than customized computer-assisted massive constructs, as they adapt to all sorts of defects in terms of sizes and shapes. Animal models using the induced membrane procedure were used to analyze the osteogenic potential of such constructs seeded with autologous MSCs.

Preliminary evaluation in subcutaneous model in sheep A sheep subcutaneous model using the induced membrane technique was set up to assess the osteogenic potential of bone constructs of clinical relevant sizes: granular and massive bone constructs exhibited bone formation after 2 months, albeit extent of bone formation was limited when compared with bone constructs implanted into bone metatarsal defects.[9,19] As observed in former femoral and tibial implantations in sheep, *Porites* scaffolds showed faster resorption compared with *Acropora* scaffolds.[9,20] Interestingly, in this animal model, preliminary experiments using MSC expressing enhanced green fluorescent protein (e-GFP) to track the fate of transplanted cells, revealed that MSC did survive and formed new bone (**Fig. 4**).

Preclinical evaluation in a bone metatarsal critical size defect model in sheep Evaluation of bone constructs combining coraline *Porites* granular (3 × 3-mm cubes) scaffolds with autologous MSCs has been performed in a bone metatarsal CSD in sheep.[21] Briefly, a 25-mm long mid-diaphyseal bone resection of the left metatarsus was created and filled with a cement spacer for 6 weeks. At that time, the cement was carefully removed through an incision made along the

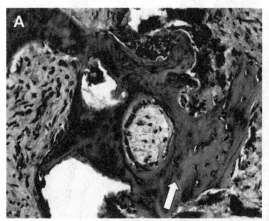
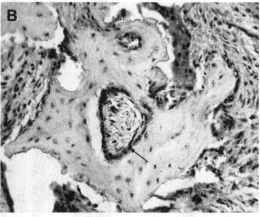

x20

Fig. 4. Immunohistochemical staining (*B*) of a decalcified section (*A*) of a massive construct seeded with autologous GFP-transduced MSCs 2 months after implantation in a subcutaneous pouch delineated by a PMMA-induced membrane in sheep. Bone formation (*white arrow*) and osteoblasts expressing eGFP (*black arrow*) are observed. The stain used for the histology (*A*) was hematoxylin-eosin-saffron (HES).

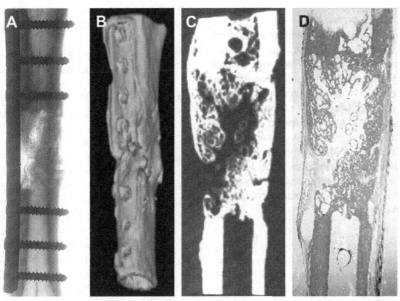

Fig. 5. Representative radiogram (*A*) and 3-dimensional tomodensitometry reconstruction (*B*), of a 25-mm-long metatarsal critical size defect of a sheep implanted with MSCs/coral constructs, 6 months after cement removal. Microradiography (*C*), and histology (*D*) of a representative 2-dimensional section were performed at that time point. The histologic stain used was von Gieson picro-fushine.

formed encapsulation membrane surrounding the cement, and the resultant cavities were either left empty (Group 1) or filled with an implant as follows: (1) plain coral scaffolds; (2) coral scaffolds loaded with MSCs; (3) autogenic, corticocancellous graft. For each animal, coral scaffolds were seeded with autologous sheep MSCs, and grown in the bioreactor for 10 days before being implanted in the donor animal. Each animal received on average 138 ± 22 pieces of Coral/MSC constructs and 8.28 ± 1.32 × 10⁶ cells/per defect.

Bone formation in the defects was analyzed for each animal at the time they were humanely killed, 6 months after the second procedure. At 6 months, unfilled defects did not heal and had characteristics of atrophic bone union, thus validating creation of a CSD. Bone deposition in the defect was minimal (≤10% of defect volume) and confined to the immediate vicinity of the proximal and distal ends of the ostectomy, where it sealed the medullary canals. Bone union was systematically achieved when defects were filled with autografts, a result that confirmed that bone healing could be achieved consistently when an appropriate material is used to fill the defect (**Fig. 3**). No significant differences were found to exist between the amount of newly formed bone present in defects filled with coral/MSCs (**Fig. 5**) and those filled with autografts (**Fig. 6**). Yet radiological scores differed significantly between defects filled with coral/MSCs

and those filled with autograft (respectively 21% and 100% healed cortices).

This study on a clinically relevant animal model thus provided the first evidence that standardized particulate bone constructs can be used to efficiently repair large bone defects using the induced membrane procedure and that the osteogenic ability of these constructs approaches partially that of bone autografts, the bone repair benchmark. Yet important parameters, such as the rate of scaffold resorption and the number of MSCs to be seeded on the scaffolds, need to be optimized before reaching pertinent definitive conclusions.

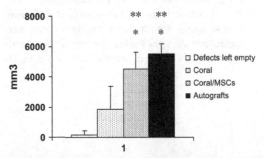

Fig. 6. Quantification of bone formation. *$P<.05$ compared with defects left empty. **$P<.05$ compared with defect filled with coral alone.

SUMMARY

The technique of the induced membrane resulted in induction of a membrane in both ectopic and or-thotopic implantation sites in several animal models. In some of these, the polymeric spacer facilitated secondary bone grafting in a manner similar to that observed in human clinical cases.

Animal experiments have provided evidence that the membrane has structural characteristics and biologic properties that may be used for bone tissue engineering purposes. It provides in particular a unique opportunity to study the effect of bone constructs engineered from granules in a controlled environment.

REFERENCES

1. de Boer HH, Wood MB. Bone changes in the vascular-ised fibular graft. J Bone Joint Surg Br 1989;71:374–8.
2. Han CS, Wood MB, Bishop AT, et al. Vascularized bone transfer. J Bone Joint Surg Am 1992;74:1441–9.
3. May JW Jr, Jupiter JB, Weiland AJ, et al. Clinical classification of post-traumatic tibial osteomyelitis. J Bone Joint Surg Am 1989;71:1422–8.
4. Masquelet AC. Muscle reconstruction in reconstruc-tive surgery: soft tissue repair and long bone recon-struction. Langenbecks Arch Surg 2003;388:344–6.
5. Masquelet AC, Fitoussi F, Begue T, et al. Recon-struction of the long bones by the induced membrane and spongy autograft. Ann Chir Plast Esthet 2000;45:346–53.
6. Klaue K, Knothe U, Masquelet AC. Effet biologique des membranes à corps étranger induites in situ sur la consolidation de greffes d'os spongieux. In: Proceedings from the 70th Réunion annuelle de la SOFCOT, p. 109–10. Paris, 1995 [in French].
7. Pelissier P, Masquelet AC, Bareille R, et al. Induced membranes secrete growth factors including vascular and osteoinductive factors and could stimu-late bone regeneration. J Orthop Res 2004;22:73–9.
8. Viateau V, Guillemin G, Yang YC, et al. A technique for creating critical-size defects in the metatarsus of sheep for use in investigation of healing of long-bone defects. Am J Vet Res 2004;65:1653–7.
9. Bensidhoum M, Viateau V, Guillemin G, et al. A novel animal model for studying the bone formation capacity of stem cell loaded biomaterials. Proceed-ings from the TERMIS EU June 22–26th, 2008, Porto.
10. Hurley LA, Stinchfield FE, Basset CAL, et al. The role of soft tissues in osteogenesis. J Bone Joint Surg Am 1959;41:1243–66.
11. Freund R, Wolff TW, Freund B. Silicone block inter-position for traumatic bone loss. Orthopedics 2000;23:802–4.
12. Abbondanzo SL, Young VL, Wei MQ, et al. Silicone gel-filled breast and testicular implant capsules: a histologic and immunophenotypic study. Mod Pathol 1999;12:706–13.
13. Smith RJ, Atkinson RE, Jupiter JB. Silicone synovitis of the wrist. J Hand Surg Am 1985;10:47–60.
14. Pap G, Machner A, Rinnert T, et al. Development and characteristics of a synovial-like interface membrane around cemented tibial hemiarthroplas-ties in a novel rat model of aseptic prosthesis loos-ening. Arthritis Rheum 2001;44:956–63.
15. Togawa D, Bauer TW, Lieberman IH, et al. Histologic evaluation of human vertebral bodies after vertebral augmentation with polymethyl methacrylate. Spine 2003;28:1521–7.
16. Salmon R, Duncan W. Determination of the critical size for non healing defects in the mandibular bone of sheep. Part 1: a pilot study. J N Z Soc Perio-dontol 1997;81:6–15.
17. Gugala Z, Gogolewski S. Regeneration of segmental diaphyseal defects in sheep tibiae using resorbable polymeric membranes: a preliminary study. J Orthop Trauma. 1999;13:187–95.
18. Pélissier P, Lefèvre Y, Delmond S, et al. Influences of induced membranes on heterotopic bone formation within an osteo-inductive complex. Experimental study in rabbits. Annales de chirurgie plastique esthétique 2009;54(1):16–20 [in French].
19. David B, Bensidhoum M, Bossis D, et al. Evalua-tion of the influence of the density of mesenchy-meal stem cells seeded on coralline scaffolds on bone formation after implantation in sheep. Proceedings from the TERMIS EU June 22–26th, 2008, Porto.
20. Guillemnin G, Meunier A, Dallant P, et al. Compar-ison of coral resorption and bone apposition with two natural corals of different porosities. J Biomed Mater Res 1989;23:765–79.
21. Viateau V, Guillemin G, Bousson V, et al. Long-bone critical-size defects treated with tissue-engineered grafts: a study on sheep. J Orthop Res 2007;25(6): 741–9.

Biological Rationale for the Intramedullary Canal as a Source of Autograft Material

David J. Hak, MD, MBA[a],*, Jason L. Pittman, MD, PhD[b]

KEYWORDS
- Autogenous bone graft • Intramedullary bone graft harvest
- Reamer irrigator aspirator • Growth factors
- Bone formation

The iliac crest has long been considered to be the gold standard donor site for harvesting autogenous bone for use in situations requiring a biologically active bone graft. Complications and morbidity associated with autogenous iliac crest bone grafting is well documented.[1] Several decades ago surgeons suggested the use of bone debris obtained from reaming of the intramedullary canal of long bones as an alternative source of autogenous bone graft material.[2–4] With standard reamers, bone graft may be extracted from the intramedullary canal as the reamer is pulled out of the bone, and some additional graft may be recovered from the flutes of the reamer heads. Although in these reports the use of bone graft harvested by intramedullary reaming was successful, there has been no direct clinical comparison of bone graft material harvested from the intramedullary canal with that harvested from the iliac crest.

The Reamer-Irrigator-Aspirator (RIA, Synthes, Paoli, PA) was initially designed to decrease embolic complications associated with standard reaming; however, clinicians quickly capitalized on its ability to harvest a large quantity of autogenous bone graft.[5] Using the RIA, graft material is removed from the canal by continuous suction and irrigation. Corticocancellous bone and other particulate debris can be harvested with a simple in-line filter system. In addition, a large volume of aspirate, including the irrigation fluid, is collected in a separate container. Compared with a standard reamer, the RIA device offers a much more efficient technique for harvesting material from the intramedullary canal. The biologic potential of bone harvested from the intramedullary canal with standard reamers has been previously studied, and with the advent of the use of RIA there has been renewed interest in exploring the biologic properties of this graft source.

Iliac crest bone graft is considered the gold standard because it is known to be osteogenic, osteoconductive, and osteoinductive. To be osteogenic, a bone graft substance must contain viable osteoblasts or stem cells that can differentiate along the bone-forming lineage. To be osteoconductive, the material must have a 3-dimensional architecture that promotes bone formation. Finally, to be osteoinductive, the substance must contain bone morphogenic proteins. For bone harvested from intramedullary reaming to serve as an alternative graft source it must possess these same properties.

CELLULAR CONTENT OF INTRAMEDULLARY REAMINGS

The intramedullary canal contains bone marrow and vasculature that make up two microenvironments

a Department of Orthopedic Surgery, Denver Health/University of Colorado, 777 Bannock Street, MC 0188, Denver, CO 80204, USA
b Department of Orthopedic Surgery, Boston University School of Medicine, Boston, MA, USA
* Corresponding author.
E-mail address: david.hak@dhha.org (D.J. Hak).

Orthop Clin N Am 41 (2010) 57–61
doi:10.1016/j.ocl.2009.07.005

or "niches," termed the vascular and osteoblastic "niches."[6] Most stem cells found in the bone marrow are hematopoietic stem cells (HSC), whereas the smaller population of stem cells are the mesenchymal stem cells (MSC).[6]

The Osteoblastic Niche

One population of HSCs is found lining the endosteal bone in close proximity to osteoblasts, which suggests a close relationship between hematopoiesis and osteogenesis. A significant function of the osteoblastic niche is to support the HSCs and hematopoiesis. When bone marrow is transplanted into an irradiated organism, it is necessary for osteoblasts to be present to obtain a successful grafting of the transplanted marrow.[6] The osteoblastic niche is responsible for providing the signals that regulate the population of HSCs in undifferentiated states.[7] Of these signals, bone morphogenic protein (BMP) and parathyroid hormone (PTH) are key proteins that regulate the formation of osteoblastic cells lining trabecular bone.

The Vascular Niche

The vascular niche of the intramedullary bone marrow provides a pathway for the mature hemopoietic cells generated in the osteoblastic niche to reach the peripheral circulation through the fenestrated walls of the bone marrow sinusoids.[6,7] Within the vascular niche, a cell line of mesenchymal origin is found surrounding and in direct contact with the endothelial cells of the microvasculature. Because of the rich intramedullary blood supply, bone harvested from the intramedullary canal may contain a larger quantity of blood vessel fragments and thus a greater number of these MSCs than bone harvested from the iliac crest.

Pericytes are distinct, polymorphic cells that have multiple, branching cytoplasmic processes that encircle the microvascular capillary.[8–10] There is evidence to suggest that the pericyte acts as a osteoblast progenitor cell when stimulated in vitro; however, it is not clear under what circumstances the pericyte will go down this particular differentiation pathway in situ.[10]

Doherty and colleagues[10] placed isolated pericytes in a diffusion chamber and followed their differentiation and showed that the pericytes expressed markers that are indicative of osteoblast formation (osteopontin, osteonectin, bone sialoprotein, and osteocalcin). The high levels of osteopontin secreted at the onset of mineralization detected within the diffusion chamber have been shown in other studies to be indicative of mature osteoblast formation.

Brighton and colleagues[8] showed that pericytes differentiated down the osteoblastic pathway and synthesized an increased amount of alkaline phosphatase (2–3 times greater) when placed under low oxygen tension (3%) conditions versus 21% to 60% oxygen.

VARIATION IN CELLULAR CONTENT BASED ON HARVEST LOCATION

Although the iliac crest has long been the gold standard, it is not because the bone harvested from this site has been identified as superior. In fact, there is some variation in the population of stem cells among different bone sites, and alternative bone graft donor sites may offer higher concentrations of various stem cell populations.

Investigators have studied the use of bone marrow aspiration from the vertebral body as an alternative to the iliac crest. In a clinical study of 21 adults undergoing posterior spinal fixation, McLain and colleagues[11] found that transpedicular aspirates of vertebral bone marrow had greater concentrations of progenitor cells compared with matched controls from the iliac crest. In a similar study, investigators studied bone marrow harvested from the vertebral body and iliac crest of 15 adults undergoing both anterior and posterior spinal surgery.[12] Progenitor cells from the vertebral body exhibited an increased level of alkaline phosphatase activity. Higher numbers of proliferating colonies of cells that promote osteogenesis were found in the vertebral body aspirates compared with the iliac crest aspirates. Progenitor cells from both sites expressed comparable levels of CD166, CD105, CD49a, and CD63 cell surface receptors.

GROWTH FACTOR CONTENT OF INTRAMEDULLARY REAMINGS

In a direct comparison between iliac crest and intramedullary reamings, Schmidmaier and colleagues[13] determined that reaming debris contains comparable quantities of growth factors as iliac crest. In addition, the aspirated irrigation fluid also contains growth factors. The growth factors (BMP-2, BMP-4, transforming growth factor [TGF]-β1, insulin-like growth factor-I (IGF-I), fibroblastic growth factor-a (FGFa), fibroblastic growth factor-b (FGFb), platelet-derived growth factor-bb (PDGFbb), and vascular endothelial growth factor [VEGF]) were quantified by enzyme-linked immunosorbent assay (ELISA) assay and then normalized by the weight of the harvested bony material. BMP-4 was not detected in material taken from either the iliac crest or the

RIA reaming debris. However, five growth factors (BMP-2, TGF-β1, IGF-I, FGFa, and PDGFbb) were found to be higher in the RIA reaming debris compared with iliac crest curettings. Not only were five of the quantified growth factors found to be higher in the RIA reaming debris than in the iliac crest graft material, but the total protein was found to be 2.1 times higher in the RIA reaming debris. Iliac crest had higher levels of VEGF and FGFb than the RIA reaming debris.[13] Although this study did quantify the various growth factors present in RIA reaming debris and in the RIA aspiration fluid, the study did not specifically examine their osteoinductive capacity.

VIABILITY OF MATERIAL FROM INTRAMEDULLARY REAMING

Investigators have raised concern about the cellular viability of bone grafts harvested by intramedullary reaming secondary to the heat that can be generated during the reaming process.[14–20] Thermally induced osteonecrosis not only injures the cortical bone and cells, but it can also denature critical proteins necessary for stimulating bone growth.

Necrosis of bone can occur at a temperature of 46°C following an exposure time of 5 minutes. The small vessels coursing through bone are even more heat sensitive than bone tissue, and thermal damage to the blood vessels can impair the nutrition of the bone.[21] Using specific investigation methods, others have found that the threshold value of thermal osteonecrosis was 47°C with an exposure time of 1 minute.[22]

The design of intramedullary reamers has evolved from early designs with shallow flutes to contemporary designs with deep flutes and narrow drive shafts. Although this evolution occurred to minimize pressure build up during reaming, it also results in decreased temperature elevation that can be seen with older reamer designs. Significant heat generation is possible in certain circumstances that may lead to thermal bone necrosis. Because of the continuous irrigation, and the sharp single-use reamer cutting head, heat build up with the RIA system is substantially less than with conventional reaming. Higgins and colleagues[23] reported that the maximum temperatures reached in the distal diaphysis in the RIA group (42.0 ± 9.1°C) were significantly lower ($P = .025$) than in the standard reaming group (58.7 ± 15.9°C).

BIOLOGIC ACTIVITY OF REAMING DEBRIS HARVESTED WITH STANDARD REAMERS

Tydings and colleagues[24] reported their findings that human reaming debris continued to calcify when implanted into a rat muscle pouch. These results led them to speculate that intramedullary canal reamings may be a superior bone graft material. In a study by Frölke and colleagues,[25] bone graft was obtained from the iliac crest and from femoral intramedullary reaming of sheep and grown in cell culture. Cell viability was determined by measuring the activity of alkaline phosphatase. Iliac crest and cortical reamings were found to have similar osteoblastic properties as determined by the response to vitamin D stimulation. In a subsequent study, Frölke and colleagues[26] compared femoral reaming debris with iliac crest graft in a sheep tibial osteotomy model. The osteotomy site was distracted 5 mm and the tibia stabilized with an external fixator. The use of reaming debris produced a comparable volume of callus formation at time points 3, 4, and 6 weeks.[26]

Wenisch and colleagues[27] determined that bone graft obtained from intramedullary reaming contained multipotent stem cells. In this study, intramedullary reamings were obtained from 12 patients undergoing reamed intramedullary nailing for closed diaphyseal fractures. These cells were cultured and characterized according to morphology, proliferative capacity, cell surface antigens, and differentiation capacity. Investigators found that the cells differentiated along the osteogenic pathway. Histologically, the reaming debris was found to have bony fragments that ranged in size from 0.2 to 2.0 mm in length. Under light microscopy, the bone fragments appeared to be intact. Under transmission electron microscopic examination, many altered cells were found along the external surfaces of the bony fragments.[27] The destruction of the cellular structures along the external surfaces of the bony fragments observed in the reaming debris could explain the large increase in the quantity of growth factors detected in reaming debris versus material obtained from the iliac crest.[13] However, when the cells derived from reaming debris were analyzed by flow cytometry for viability, greater than 95% of the cell population was found to have remained viable following intramedullary reaming using a traditional reaming device.[27] However, under conditions of excessive reaming, the vitality of reaming debris is destroyed.[28]

BIOLOGIC ACTIVITY OF REAMING DEBRIS HARVESTED WITH THE REAMER-IRRIGATOR-ASPIRATOR

Hammer and colleagues[29] examined the use of bone graft harvested with RIA in a sheep tibial defect model. An 8-mm segmental defect was created at the mid-diaphysis of sheep tibia and the wound closed. The medullary cavity was then reamed to 11 mm with either a standard reamer or RIA. Reamings from the different devices were allowed to naturally disperse into the defect in two groups of animals. In a third group the defect site was opened and the additional reaming debris harvested by the RIA device was applied to the defect site. All animals then had an intramedullary tibial nail placed. At 6 weeks they found significant improvement in the size and strength of the callus in animals in which the captured RIA reamings were placed into the bone defect.

The osteogenic potential of fluid aspirate obtained using the RIA system was evaluated by Porter and colleagues.[30] Aspirate was obtained during the reaming of the upper half of the femoral canal during hip arthroplasty in five patients. The aspirate was filtered to remove osseous particles and then the filtrate processed by centrifugation to isolate the cellular components. An average of 230 mL of material was retrieved with an average of 6.2×10^6 nucleated cells per milliliter of aspirate. They found that the aqueous supernatant contained FGF-2, IGF-1, and latent TGF-β1, but that BMP-2 was below the limit for detection. Cells present in the fluid included fibroblastic cells that displayed a surface marker profile consistent with mesenchymal stem cells. These cells could be induced to differentiate along osteogenic, adipogenic, and chondrogenic lines. The authors suggested that the ideal graft would be a combination of the osseous particles, providing an osteoconductive scaffold for bone growth, and the cellular material in the filtrate, providing the osteogenic properties for bone regeneration.

VOLUME OF BONE GRAFT REQUIRED

In the literature, there is little information about the minimal volume of bone graft needed to successfully heal a specific size defect.[31] Clinically, the amount of autogenous bone available from a standard iliac crest bone graft is not always sufficient for large segmental bone defects. In these situations, surgeons have suggested the use of various bone graft substitutes as an extender for the autogenous bone graft. The large volume of bone graft that can be obtained with RIA is likely beneficial when treating very large bone defects. On average, roughly 70 mL of bone graft can be obtained from the femur using RIA, which is far greater than can be routinely obtained from the iliac crest.

SUMMARY

Although no single study has compared bone graft harvested with the RIA to iliac crest bone graft, studies have shown that material harvested by RIA fulfills all the requirements to be equivalent to the gold standard. The RIA graft contains stem cells that can differentiate along the bone-forming lineage, therefore it offers osteogenic properties. Although morselized, the material still likely provides some 3-dimensional properties similar to the trabecular bone harvested from the iliac crest. Finally, several studies have shown the presence of bone morphogenetic proteins that are osteoinductive in both the bone graft material and fluid aspirate obtained with RIA.

Future basic science and clinical studies will better elucidate the potential for bone graft harvested by RIA to solve difficult bone-healing problems. The potential for concentration and injection of the aspirate fluid has yet to be explored. For many surgeons, the ability to harvest a large quantity of bone in a minimally invasive manner currently offers an important clinical benefit for the management of difficult nonunions and large bone defects.

REFERENCES

1. Goulet JA, Senunas LE, DeSilva GL, et al. Autogenous iliac crest bone graft. Complications and functional assessment. Clin Orthop Relat Res 1997; 339:76–81.
2. Alfred R, Tydings J, Martino L, et al. Intramedullary bone reamings augmenting fracture fixation. Surg Forum 1984;35:523–5.
3. Chapman MW. Closed intramedullary bone grafting and nailing of segmental defects of the femur. A report of three cases. J Bone Joint Surg Am 1980; 62:1004–8.
4. Chapman MW. Closed intramedullary bone grafting for diaphyseal defects of the femur. Instr Course Lect 1983;32:317–24.
5. Newman JT, Stahel PF, Smith WR, et al. A new minimally invasive technique for large volume bone graft harvest for treatment of fracture nonunions. Orthopaedics 2008;31(3):257–61.
6. Yin T, Li L. The stem cell niches in bone. J Clin Invest 2006;116:1195–201.
7. Kopp HG, Avecilla ST, Hooper AT, et al. The bone marrow vascular niche: home of HSC differentiation and mobilization. Physiology Bethesda 2005;20: 349–56.
8. Brighton CT, Lorich DG, Kupcha R, et al. The pericyte as a possible osteoblast progenitor cell. Clin Orthop Relat Res 1992;275:287–99.
9. Schor AM, Allen TD, Canfield AE, et al. Pericytes derived from the retinal microvasculature undergo calcification in vitro. J Cell Sci 1990;97:449–61.
10. Doherty MJ, Ashton BA, Walsh S, et al. Vascular pericytes express osteogenic potential in vitro and in vivo. J Bone Miner Res 1998;13:828–38.

11. McLain RF, Fleming JE, Boehm CA, et al. Aspiration of osteoprogenitor cells for augmenting spinal fusion: comparison of progenitor cell concentrations from the vertebral body and iliac crest. J Bone Joint Surg Am 2005;87:2655–61.

12. Risbud MV, Shapiro IM, Guttapalli A, et al. Osteogenic potential of adult human stem cells of the lumbar vertebral body the iliac crest. Spine 2006; 31:83–9.

13. Schmidmaier G, Herrmann S, Green J, et al. Quantitative assessment of growth factors in reaming aspirate, iliac crest, and platelet preparation. Bone 2006;39:1156–63.

14. Frölke JP, Peters R, Boshuizen K, et al. The assessment of cortical heat during intramedullary reaming of long bones. Injury 2001;32:683–8.

15. García OGR, Mombiela FL, De La Fuente CJ, et al. The influence of the size and condition of the reamers on bone temperature during intramedullary reaming. J Bone Joint Surg Am 2004;86-A: 994–9.

16. Giannoudis PV, Snowden S, Matthews SJ, et al. Temperature rise during reamed tibial nailing. Clin Orthop Relat Res 2002;395:255–61.

17. Karunakar MA, Frankenburg EP, Le TT, et al. The thermal effects of intramedullary reaming. J Orthop Trauma 2004;18:674–9.

18. Leunig M, Hertel R. Thermal necrosis after tibial reaming for intramedullary nail fixation: a report of three cases. J Bone Joint Surg Br 1996;78: 584–7.

19. Ochsner PE, Baumgart F, Kohler G. Heat-induced segmental necrosis after reaming of one humeral and two tibial fractures with a narrow medullary canal. Injury 1998;29(Suppl 2):B1–10.

20. Mueller CA, Rahn BA. Intramedullary pressure increase and increase in cortical temperature during reaming of the femoral medullary cavity: the effect of draining the medullary contents before reaming. J Trauma 2003;55:495–503.

21. Lundskog J. Heat and bone tissue: an experimental investigation of the thermal properties of bone tissue and threshold levels for thermal injury. Scand J Plast Reconstr Surg 1972;9:1–80.

22. Eriksson AR, Albrektsson T. Temperature threshold levels for heat induced bone tissue injury: a vital-microscopic study in the rabbit. J Prosthet Dent 1983;50:101–7.

23. Higgins TF, Casey V, Bachus K. Cortical heat generation using an irrigating/aspirating single-pass reaming vs. conventional stepwise reaming. J Orthop Trauma 2007;21:192–7.

24. Tydings JD, Martino LJ, Kircher M, et al. Viability of intramedullary canal bone reamings for continued calcification. Am J Surg 1987;153:306–9.

25. Frölke JPM, Nulend JK, Semeins CM, et al. Viable osteoblastic potential of cortical reamings from intramedullary nailing. J Orthop Res 2004;22:1271–5.

26. Frölke JPM, Bakker FC, Patka P, et al. Reaming debris in osteotomized sheep tibiae. J Trauma 2001;50:65–70.

27. Wenisch S, Trinkaus K, Hild A, et al. Human reaming debris: a source of multipotent stem cells. Bone 2005;36:74–83.

28. Hoegel F, Mueller CA, Peter R, et al. Bone debris: dead matter or vital osteoblasts. J Trauma 2004; 56:363–7.

29. Hammer TO, Wieling R, Green JM, et al. Effect of re-implanted particles from intramedullary reaming on mechanical properties and callus formation. A laboratory study. J Bone Joint Surg Br 2007;89(11): 1534–8.

30. Porter RM, Liu F, Pilapil C, et al. Osteogenic potential of reamer irrigator aspirator (RIA) aspirate collected from patients undergoing hip arthroplasty. J Orthop Res 2009;27(1):42–9.

31. DeVries WJ, Runyon CL, Martinez SA, et al. Effect of volume variations on osteogenic capabilities of autogenous cancellous bone graft in dogs. Am J Vet Res 1996;57:1501–5.

Treatment of Large Segmental Bone Defects with Reamer-Irrigator-Aspirator Bone Graft: Technique and Case Series

Todd A. McCall, MD[a], David S. Brokaw, MD[b],
Bradley A. Jelen, DO[b], D. Kevin Scheid, MD[b],
Angela V. Scharfenberger, MD[c], Dean C. Maar, MD[b],
James M. Green, BS[d], Melanie R. Shipps, BS[b],
Marcus B. Stone, PhD[e], Dana Musapatika, MS, MSc[f],
Timothy G. Weber, MD[b],*

KEYWORDS

- RIA • Bone graft • Growth factors • Reaming
- Segmental fractures

Treatment of large segmental bone defects is a difficult challenge for orthopedic surgeons. These large defects can be caused by traumatic injury or surgical treatment of infection or tumors. Historically, amputation was the best option for many of these patients, but limb salvage has become more common. Review of available literature demonstrates that several treatment modalities have had some success in treating segmental bone defects:

> Ilizarov bone transport
> Autogenous cortical or cancellous bone graft
> Vascularized fibula graft
> Recombinant bone morphogenic protein
> Calcium phosphate fillers[1–20]

Autogenous bone graft has been the gold standard for bone graft. It is osteogenic, osteoinductive, and osteoconductive. When the defect is large, however, the traditional supply of autogenous graft may not be sufficient. There can be significant morbidity with harvesting large quantities of bone. Many studies show high incidences of complications from iliac crest harvest, including donor site pain and injury to cutaneous nerves resulting in painful neuromas.[21–24] With the recent availability of bone morphogenic protein (BMPs), many surgeons have decreased their use of autogenous bone graft to avoid potential complications at the donor site. Although there are several studies that show BMP is effective for nonunions and healing cortical defects,[1,15,17,18] its high cost

---

[a] Orthopedic Clinics of Daytona Beach, 1075 Mason Avenue, Daytona Beach, FL 32117, USA
[b] OrthoIndy, 1801 North Senate Boulevard, # 200, Indianapolis, IN 46202, USA
[c] University Orthopedic Consultants, Suite 1002 College Plaza, 8215 112th Street, Edmonton, T6G2C8 Alberta, Canada
[d] Synthes, Post Office Box 1766, 1690 Russell Road, Paoli, PA 19301, USA
[e] Alegius Consulting, 1203 Lexington Woods Drive, Avon, IN 46123, USA
[f] Synthes, 1301 Goshen Parkway, West Chester, PA 19380, USA
* Corresponding author.
E-mail address: dmusapatika@orthoindy.com (T.G. Weber).

Orthop Clin N Am 41 (2010) 63–73
doi:10.1016/j.ocl.2009.08.002
0030-5898/09/$ – see front matter © 2010 Elsevier Inc. All rights reserved.

may be prohibitive at some institutions, especially in very large defects, where a large quantity of graft would be needed.

Bone grafting of defects often is delayed after primary internal fixation to allow soft tissue healing, decrease infection risk, and prevent graft resorption during the early inflammatory healing phase. Cement spacers with antibiotics can be used to temporarily fill defects. This has many advantages. Cement can give structural support and decrease implant loading. It maintains a void that allows easy placement of graft and provides local antibiotics in areas of open fractures at high risk for infection. Cement spacers also induce formation of pseudosynovial membrane, which creates a contained defect for bone grafting.[25] This membrane has been shown to produce growth factors and osteoinductive factors including BMP-2.[26]

The reamer-irrigator-aspirator (RIA) originally was designed as a single-pass intramedullary reamer that creates a negative pressure within the canal in an effort to decrease pulmonary insult from marrow contents during the course of reaming for femur fractures. RIA has several unique characteristics allowing it to achieve this result. The reamer head is extremely sharp. It is a single-use reamer that allows reaming to a premeasured diameter with a single pass, as opposed to sequential passes with incrementally larger reamers. It also has both an irrigation and aspiration port. Irrigation of the canal with normal saline during the reaming process decreases the overall temperature within the canal and assists in the aspiration process, as it decreases the viscosity of the intramedullary contents. Aspiration allows for removal of reaming debris and creates constant negative pressure in the canal. RIA has been used to debride the intramedullary canal for treatment of bone infections. It also can be modified by placing a screen trap in line with the aspiration port to capture the bone debris aspirated from the medullary canal in a sterile fashion.

The ideal treatment for large segmental defects of long bones would be inexpensive, have minimal adverse effects, be effective at obtaining union, and provide enough graft volume to fill the defect. The intramedullary canal of femurs and tibias is relatively easy to access and contains large amounts of cancellous bone graft. Intramedullary reamings have been shown to have viable cells capable of new osteosynthesis.[27–29] Recent quantitative analysis found higher levels of fibroblast growth factor (FGFa), platelet-derived growth factor (PDGF), insulinlike growth factor (IGF)-1, BMP-2, and transforming growth factor (TGF)-β1 in RIA bone graft compared with iliac crest bone graft.[30] This study is designed to evaluate the efficacy of healing and associated complications in patients with large segmental defects treated with bone graft obtained by RIA.

MATERIALS AND METHODS

This prospective study was conducted between February 2003 and March 2007. Investigators obtained institutional review board approval and written informed consent from all patients. Twenty one patients, 13 male and 8 female, with an average age of 30.6 years, with segmental bone defects agreed to participate. The defect size ranged from 2 to 14.5 cm (average 6.6 cm). Three patients had at least one surgical procedure at an outside hospital. All subsequent surgeries were performed by fellowship-trained orthopedic trauma surgeons at a level 1 trauma center. Eight patients smoked, and 13 did not. Mechanism of injury included nine motorcycle collisions, five motor vehicle collisions, four gun shot wounds, one car versus pedestrian, one car versus bicyclist, and one crush injury. There were 5 femurs, 15 tibias and 1 ulna treated. The average time from initial injury to RIA procedure was 141 days (range 31 to 582 days).

All patients with open fractures were treated with appropriate surgical debridements and antibiotics. **Box 1** outlines the treatment algorithm. An average of 4.8 procedures were performed at the defect site before placement of bone graft. The 20 open fractures were classified as 8 grade 3A, 9 grade 3B, and 2 grade 3C. Eight patients needed soft tissue flap coverage, including three free flaps and five local flaps. Eighteen patients had antibiotic spacers placed into the defect site before bone grafting. The RIA graft was obtained from 21 femurs and 2 tibias. One patient had bone graft harvested from both the contralateral tibia and femur, and another had bone harvested from the ipsilateral femur and contralateral tibia. Filtered bone graft volume was measured in 19 patients. The amount of bone graft harvested was not maximized in patients with smaller defects.

Surgical Technique

After induction of general anesthesia, the patients were positioned supine on a radiolucent table. The defect site was prepared first to ensure that there was no sign of infection and to limit the time span that the graft was exposed out of the body. An appropriate skin incision was made depending on location of the defect and previous incisions. In cases with PMMA spacers, the pseudomembrane enveloping the spacer was incised longitudinally to allow for closure after grafting. The

Box 1
Treatment algorithms

Open Fractures

↓

Antibiotics in emergency room

↓

Urgent irrigation and debridements (I&D) in operating room with removal of devascularized soft tissue and bone

Internal or External Fixation

Plus or minus VAC dressing

↓

Repeat I&Ds until wound clean and all devitalized tissue removed

↓

Definitive fixation with plate or nail if previously ex fixed

Wound closed or covered with flap

Antibiotic cement spacer placed into defect

↓

Incisions and soft tissues allowed to heal (4 to 6 weeks)

↓

Psuedomembrane incised and cement spacer removed

Fibrous tissue debrided from defect if polymethylmethacrylate (PMMA) spacer not used

Medullary canal opened

Defect grafted with RIA bone graft if no sign of infection

Weight bearing limited until radiographic consolidation

spacer was removed and the bone edges cleaned of interposed fibrous tissue.

When graft was harvested from the femur, a bump was placed under the ipsilateral pelvis similar to position for free leg femoral nail. The narrowest section of the femur or tibia was templated on anterior–posterior (AP) and lateral fluoroscopy to determine the intramedullary canal size (**Fig. 1**). Reamer size then was chosen to be approximately 1 to 1.5 mm larger than the determined canal size. A percutaneous technique was used to locate the piriformis fossa or lateral starting point at the tip of the greater trochanter. This was verified with biplanar fluoroscopy. The standard entry point for tibial intramedullary nailing was used for tibial graft harvest. A 13 mm cannulated drill bit was used to open the entry site, after which a ball tip guide rod was advanced down the canal. The Reamer Irrigator Aspirator (RIA) system (Synthes, West Chester, Pennsylvania) then was prepared to harvest bone graft (**Fig. 2**). This included attaching an appropriately sized reamer head, a 3 or 5 L saline bag to the irrigation port, suction to the aspiration port and a screen trap in line with the suction tubing. The Screen Trap (Biomet, Warsaw, Indiana) has a pore size of approximately 500 μm. Gravity flow and vacuum suction were used to maintain irrigation flow. The canal then was reamed with an appropriately sized reamer in an alternating advance-and-withdraw motion (see **Fig. 1**). The femur received two to four passes of the RIA. For larger defects, graft volume can be increased by positioning the guide rod in the lateral condyle first and then into the medial condyle to enable graft acquisition from both (**Fig. 3**). When reaming is completed, the trap is disconnected and bone graft collected. The harvested bone graft then is packed into the defect. The pseudomembrane is closed to contain the graft, and skin incisions are closed.

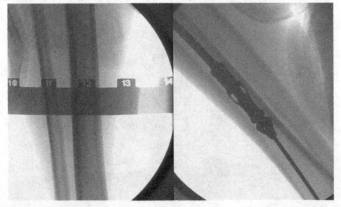

Fig. 1. Templating and reaming canal.

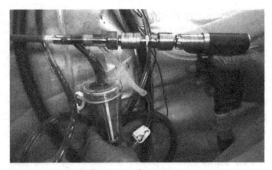

Fig. 2. Reamer-irrigator-aspirator set-up.

RESULTS
Follow-up

Twenty of the 21 patients (95%) have been followed to conclusion. Patients were followed clinically and radiographically until declared healed or failure of treatment. One patient (5%) was lost to follow-up before complete healing.

Graft Harvest

The bone graft volume was measured in 19 of the 21 patients and averaged 64 cc. Two patients had graft harvested from a femur and a tibia. As expected, tibia bone graft volume (37.5 cc) was less than femur volume (67 cc). These extracted volumes, however, were not the maximum volume of graft available. Patients with smaller defects needed less bone graft; therefore less graft was harvested.

Donor Site Complications

No patients had serious donor site morbidity. There were no donor site hematomas, infections, or fractures. No second surgeries were required at donor sites. The authors did not perform routine radiographic examinations of donor bone site. Eight patients who had antegrade femoral RIA procedures had pelvis or hip radiographs for follow-up of pelvic ring or contralateral hip injuries.

Two of these patients (25%) were noted to have Brooker class 1 heterotopic ossification in the soft tissues near the abductor insertion. None of these patients had clinical or subjective symptoms at donor site.

Defect Site Complications

Of the 20 patients followed to conclusion, 10 had no defect site complications after bone grafting. Ten patients (50%) had defect site complications. There were six deep infections and four nonunions (two with hardware failure). Four of the patients with infection and three with nonunion eventually healed the defect.

Defect healing

Twenty patients with segmental bone defects were followed to conclusion. There were 5 femurs, 14 tibias, and 1 ulna. Eighteen of these 20 patients had PMMA spacers in the defect before bone grafting. Sixteen patients were treated with plates, and 4 were treated with intramedullary (IM) nails. Seventeen of 20 patients (85%) completely healed at an average 11 months (range 2.5 to 39 months). Ten of these 17 (58%) healed with no additional surgery after RIA bone graft. Seven patients needed additional surgeries after original RIA. Two patients healed after exchange intramedullary nail; one patient developed a deep infection but healed after I&D and repeat RIA. One proximal tibia healed after revision compression plating with cancellous bone graft harvested from the distal femur, and one healed after I&D and Enders rod (West Chester, Pennsylvania) placement. One healed after repeat I&Ds, and one developed deep infection after the defect healed, requiring I&D and plate removal (**Table 1**).

Illustrative Case (1st RIA Case Performed)

A 35-year-old woman presented 6 months after a motorcycle accident with a large, open, draining wound of her tibia. After debridement of the wound

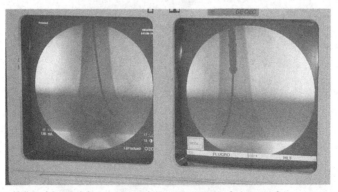

Fig. 3. Guide rod in medial and lateral femoral condyle to maximize bone graft.

Table 1
Results

Outcome	N	Comments
Healed without further surgery	10	No further surgery after RIA
Healed with further surgery	7	2 exchange intramedullary nails 1 I&D with removal of bone graft followed by repeat RIA 1 compression plate with junctional bone graft 1 I&D with Enders rod placement 1 repeat I&D for wound infection 1 deep infection after defect healed treated with I&D and hardware removal
Failed	3	2 deep infections with removal of RIA graft 1 recurrent nonunion with plate failure × 2

and bone, she had a 14 cm defect that was managed with a block of methylmethacrylate and covered with a free flap (**Fig. 4**). Eight weeks later with a stable wound, the RIA was used to harvest bone graft from the ipsilateral femur using a piriformis entry site. The bone graft was used to fill the 14 cm defect with no adjunctive materials added. Ultimately, the patient went on to union of the defect at about 10 months after bone grafting. Hardware removal was performed because of prominent hardware that was causing pain. Unfortunately, the patient fractured through the graft while snow skiing and required a replating. An attempt was made at union with casting. At the time of replating the patient did not have any formal bone grafting other than some local bone graft taken from prominent bone where the bone had grown up around the previously removed plate. Her final radiographs after replating show solid union (**Figs. 5–8**) of the tibia and recovery of the donor femur site.

Failures

Three patients were considered to be treatment failures: two deep infections requiring removal of RIA bone graft, and one recurrent nonunion with multiple hardware failures. The first failure was a male smoker with grade 3B open tibia and a 10 cm tibial defect from a motorcycle accident. The wound was contaminated with dirt and organic debris. He underwent external fixation and multiple irrigation and debridements with antibiotic spacers and required a gastrocnemius muscle flap for coverage. The defect was fixed with a locking plate, and RIA bone graft was performed at 3 months after injury. He developed wound drainage 2 weeks after operating and was treated with antibiotics. At 22 days after operating,

the patient had surgical irrigation and debridement. Much of the graft was removed, but there was a shell of cortical–cancellous bone around the periphery, which was left intact. The patient had subsequent repeat bone graft with BMP-2. He was noncompliant with intravenous antibiotic treatment and did not show up for the most recent clinic appointments. At last follow-up, he had incomplete radiographic consolidation, but clinically had minimal pain at fracture.

The second failure was another grade 3B tibia with a 10 cm defect from a motorcycle accident. The patient had external fixation of his tibia and

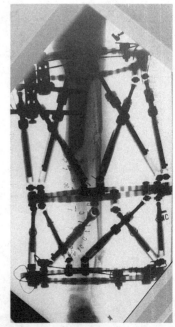

Fig. 4. Anterior–posterior radiograph showing 14 cm defect with methylmethacrylate spacer.

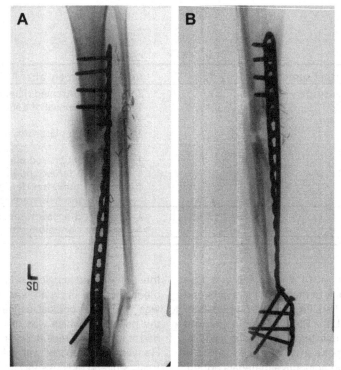

Fig. 5. Anterior–posterior (*A*) and lateral (*B*) radiographs 10 months after reamer-irrigator-aspirator bone grafting to the tibia showing union of the defect.

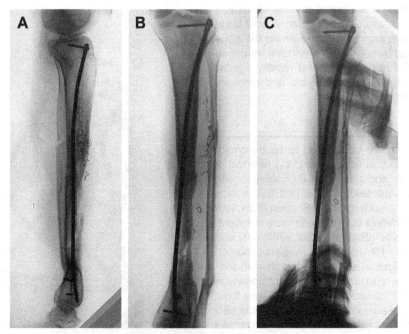

Fig. 6. Radiographs of a ununited tibial fracture from a skiing accident. Previous union attempt using a cast had failed. (*A*) Lateral view, (*B*) Anterior-posterior view, (*C*) Stress view.

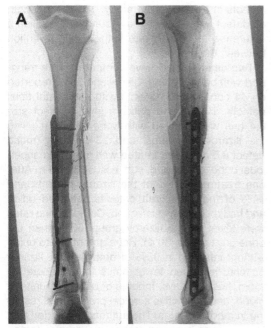

Fig. 7. Anterior posterior radiographs showing well-united tibia with no further bone grafting (*A, B*).

four I&Ds before open reduction and internal fixation with a locked plate. He then required free flap coverage. RIA bone graft procedure was performed 3 months after injury. Four months after

RIA, he developed wound dehiscence and drainage requiring surgical debridement with removal of the bone graft.

The third failure was a female smoker with a grade 3A distal femur fracture and a 3.5 cm defect. She was treated with irrigation and debridement and open reduction and internal fixation with a distal femur locking plate, followed by RIA bone grafting 1 month after injury. She progressed to full weight bearing as the defect consolidated radiographically. She developed nonunion with plate failure 5 months after injury. At the time of revision surgery, most of the defect had healed, but the proximal junction was not united. She had iliac crest bone graft and revision plate fixation. Sixteen months later, she had continued nonunion with hardware failure. She had revision of hardware with revision bone graft and BMP. Presently, she has good alignment, and the fracture appears to be healing.

DISCUSSION

The treatment method used for patients with segmental defects of long bones depends largely on the training and experience of the surgeon. There are two major treatment methods that can be used: stabilizing the bone out to length and filling in the defect, or using the Ilizarov principles to transport bone to correct the defect. Each of

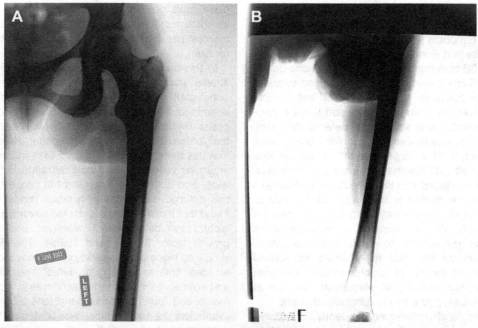

Fig. 8. (*A*) Femur donor site 6 months after reamer-irrigator-aspirator (RIA) harvest. (*B*) Femur donor site 5 years after RIA harvest.

these methods has many variations that can be used.

Review of literature of bone transport for tibial bone defects shows high healing rates but prolonged time in external fixators. Paley and Maar[7] reported 19 patients with tibial defects averaging 10 cm. They had a union rate of 100% and an external fixation index (EFI) (external fixation time [EFT] per centimeter of distraction gap) of 1.7 months per centimeter (average EFT, 17 months). A mean of 1.6 unplanned surgical procedures were performed for problems. Ten docking sites were bone grafted, and nine healed primarily. Polyzois and colleagues[31] reported on 42 patients with diaphyseal bone defects (25 tibial and 17 femoral). Preoperatively, 19 had active infection with drainage. After debridement, the mean defect was 6 cm. The mean duration of external fixation was 10 months. All patients healed, 38 without bone grafting; 4 required autogenous bone grafting. Dendrinos and colleagues[32] treated 28 tibias using the Ilizarov bone transport method. The average bone defect was 6 cm. The mean duration of treatment was 10 months. Three patients were treated with bone grafting of the docking site. Twenty-seven patients (96%) had eventual healing. There 71 minor and major complications (2.5 complications per patient), including 1 amputation. Dagher and Roukoz[33] reported on nine patients with grade 3B open tibias. Tibial defects averaged 6.3 cm and were treated with Ilizarov transport. Four patients were infected preoperatively. All nine healed with no residual infection and with less than 1 cm of leg length discrepancy (LLD). No bone graft was performed, and the EFI was 1.8 months per centimeter.

Bosse and Robb[13] reported on 16 patients with grade 3B tibia fractures. The average bone defect was 9.5 cm. External fixators were used to stabilize the fractures. Local muscle or free muscle grafts were performed to cover soft tissues. Antibiotic beads were placed in all defects. When the soft tissue was healed, the antibiotic beads were removed, and a large amount of autogenous bone graft was obtained from the posterior illiac crest and placed into the defect. All 16 fractures and defects healed at an average of 10 months. Only 6 of 16 patients healed after initial bone graft procedure. Patients required an average of six surgical procedures to achieve consolidation. The authors identified four factors associated with early failure of union: inadequate graft volume, suboptimal graft placement, infection at surgical site, and errors in surgical judgment.

Jones and colleagues[1] recently compared rBMP-2 combined with allograft bone with autogenous bone graft for reconstructing tibial cortical defects in a randomized study. The mean length of defect was 4 cm. They found no significant difference in healing rate without reintervention between the groups.

Two other authors have compared bone transport with bone grafting. Cierny and Zorn[4] reported on 44 consecutive patients with segmental tibial defects. Twenty-one patients (mean defect size 6.4 cm) were treated with bone transport using the Ilizarov apparatus, and 23 patients (mean defect 8.5 cm) were treated with massive cancellous bone grafts and soft tissue transfer. After one treatment, 71% of the Ilizarov patients and 74% of the bone graft patients achieved union and had resolution of infection. Complication rates were lower for the Ilizarov group (33%) than the bone graft group (60%). Retreatment led to union without infection in 95% of both groups. Ilizarov patients averaged fewer hours in the operating room, hospital days, months of disability, units of blood, and adjunctive surgical procedures, resulting in a cost savings. The authors concluded that Ilizarov bone transport reconstruction was faster, safer, less expensive, and easier to perform, but the final result was the same.

Green[3] retrospectively reviewed two treatment groups with bone defects: 17 patients treated by Ilizarov bone transport (mean defect 5 cm) and 15 patients treated by the Papineau bone grafting technique (mean defect 4 cm). Six of the 17 transport patients required bone grafting at the docking site to achieve union. Only two patients in the bone graft group required a second bone graft procedure. The treatment time was identical for the two groups; the EFI was 1.9 months per centimeter of defect reconstructed for both.

In this study, 18 of 20 patients had a PMMA spacer placed into the defect before the RIA bone graft procedure. This technique first was described by Masquelet, who reported on 35 cases. He described a pseudosynovial membrane that formed around the cement spacer. He stated that this membrane prevents graft resorption and improves vascularity and corticalization.[25,34] Pelissier and colleagues[26] studied the properties of this induced membrane in a rabbit model. They found that this membrane secreted several growth factors including BMP-2, vascular endothelial growth factor (VEGF), and TGFβ1. The BMP-2 level was highest at 4 weeks, which may indicate an ideal time to bone graft defect site. Viateau and colleagues studied this technique in a sheep model and found that the membrane alone was insufficient to heal critical size defects. When autologous bone graft was placed within membrane, all of the defects healed.[35]

The RIA system may have many uses, including obtaining large amounts of bone graft, debriding intramedullary infections, and reaming for intramedullary nailing. Although using RIA to obtain bone graft is a new technique, several authors previously reported on the use of intramedullary reaming material as viable bone graft.[27,29,36–39] Wenisch and colleagues[28] studied human reaming debris using cell cultures and found multipotent stem cells capable of differentiating along the osteogenic pathway. Schmidmaier and colleagues recently compared quantitative levels of growth factors from RIA aspirate, iliac crest, and platelet preparations. They found higher concentrations of five of seven growths factors (TGF-β1, IGF-I, FGFa, PDGFbb, and BMP-2) in samples obtained from intramedullary reaming debris compared with those from the iliac crest.[30]

Several recent studies have demonstrated benefits of RIA compared with traditional reaming. Husebye and colleagues[40] found that the intramedullary pressure during reaming of pig femurs was significantly lower with RIA compared with traditional reamers. Higgins and colleagues[41] showed significantly lower maximum reaming temperatures (42°C versus 58°C) with RIA compared with a traditional reamer using fresh-frozen human cadaver tibias. Pape and colleagues[42] compared traditional reamed, unreamed, and RIA-reamed femoral nailing in sheep with unilateral lung contusion. They found that the traditional reamed nail group had a higher systemic response than the RIA reamed group (higher D-dimer levels, lower polymorphonuclear neutrophils (PMN) reserve capacity, and increased pulmonary permeability).

There are very few published human data regarding the safety and efficacy of using RIA as a bone-grafting tool. Belthur and colleagues[43] recently reported the first series of prospectively monitored RIA graft patients compared with historic iliac crest bone graft (ICBG) patients. In that series, pain scores at each of the three time points—acute (less than 48 hours), intermediate (greater than 48 hours to less than 3 months), and chronic (greater than 3 months)—were significantly lower in the RIA cohort. There were no instances of numbness in the RIA group, but eight ICBG patients reported numbness. They noted two complications specifically related to RIA bone harvesting: distal perforation of the femur caused by an eccentric guide wire and an excessively anterior piriformis entry portal. Both technical errors were noted and compensated for with no final adverse effect. In this study, there were no clinically significant complications at the RIA donor site. There were no infections, no secondary surgeries, and no fractures from the use of RIA at harvest site. Two of eight patients had Brooker class 1 heterotopic ossification (HO) at the proximal femur.[44] None of these small islands of ossification in the soft tissues caused clinical or subjective symptoms. Having a small amount of HO is not unexpected given that previous studies on HO after femoral nails found incidences of 36% after reamed nails and 9% after unreamed nails.[45]

This is a report on the initial case series at the authors' institution. The authors feel that their results have improved as they learned more and improved on their operative techniques. Specifically, the authors have noted that during their early cases, they packed the graft in very tightly to maximize the amount of graft placed into the defect. During revision grafting of some of the early failures, it was found that this tightly packed graft had not consolidated. There was some peripheral revascularization and ossification, but a central core remained with a consistency similar to when it initially was placed. Although the mechanism is unclear, it appears that in later cases where the graft was not packed tightly, much faster graft incorporation and higher rate of healing of defect were obtained.

Although the authors did not have any donor site complications, there is potential for significant complications if correct technique is not used. The RIA reamers are much sharper than traditional reamers and have the potential to ream through cortical bone. The donor bone should be templated on both AP and lateral fluoroscopy, and the smaller diameter measurement should be used. Care also should be used to center the guide wire in the canal to avoid reaming eccentrically. If good technique is used, RIA is a safe technique to obtain large quantities of autogenous bone graft with minimal donor site morbidity and a high rate of defect consolidation.

REFERENCES

1. Jones AL, Bucholz RW, Bosse MJ, et al. Recombinant human BMP-2 and allograft compared with autogenous bone graft for reconstruction of diaphyseal tibial fractures with cortical defects. A randomized, controlled trial. J Bone Joint Surg Am 2006; 88(7):1431–41.

2. Finkemeier CG. Bone grafting and bone graft substitutes. J Bone Joint Surg Am 2002;84(3):454–64.

3. Green SA. Skeletal defects. A comparison of bone grafting and bone transport for segmental skeletal defects. Clin Orthop Relat Res 1994;301:111–7.

4. Cierny G 3rd, Zorn KE. Segmental tibial defects. Comparing conventional and Ilizarov methodologies. Clin Orthop Relat Res 1994;301:118–23.

5. Nusbickel FR, Dell PC, McAndrew MP, et al. Vascularized autografts for reconstruction of skeletal defects following lower extremity trauma. A review. Clin Orthop Relat Res 1989;243:65–70.

6. Nho SJ, Helfet DL, Rozbruch SR. Temporary intentional leg shortening and deformation to facilitate wound closure using the Ilizarov/Taylor spatial frame. J Orthop Trauma 2006;20(6):419–24.

7. Paley D, Maar DC. Ilizarov bone transport treatment for tibial defects. J Orthop Trauma 2000;14(2):76–85.

8. DeCoster TA, Gehlert RJ, Mikola EA, et al. Management of post-traumatic segmental bone defects. J Am Acad Orthop Surg 2004;12(1):28–38.

9. Sen C, Kocaoglu M, Eralp L, et al. Bifocal compression–distraction in the acute treatment of grade III open tibia fractures with bone and soft tissue loss: a report of 24 cases. J Orthop Trauma 2004;18(3):150–7.

10. Rozbruch SR, Weitzman AM, Watson JT, et al. Simultaneous treatment of tibial bone and soft tissue defects with the Ilizarov method. J Orthop Trauma 2006;20(3):197–205.

11. Giannikas KA, Maganaris CN, Karski MT, et al. Functional outcome following bone transport reconstruction of distal tibial defects. J Bone Joint Surg Am 2005;87(1):145–52.

12. Kocaoglu M, Eralp L, Rashid HU, et al. Reconstruction of segmental bone defects due to chronic osteomyelitis with use of an external fixator and an intramedullary nail. J Bone Joint Surg Am 2006;88(10):2137–45.

13. Bosse MJ, Robb G. Techniques for the reconstruction of large traumatic bony defects with massive autogenous cancellous bone graft. Tech Orthop 1992;7(2):17–25.

14. Enneking WF, Eady JL, Burchardt H. Autogenous cortical bone grafts in the reconstruction of segmental skeletal defects. J Bone Joint Surg Am 1980;62(7):1039–58.

15. Cook SD, Baffes GC, Wolfe MW, et al. The effect of recombinant human osteogenic protein-1 on healing of large segmental bone defects. J Bone Joint Surg Am 1994;76(6):827–38.

16. Gordon L, Chiu EJ. Treatment of infected nonunions and segmental defects of the tibia with staged microvascular muscle transplantation and bone grafting. J Bone Joint Surg Am 1988;70(3):377–86.

17. Salkeld SL, Patron LP, Barrack RL, et al. The effect of osteogenic protein-1 on the healing of segmental bone defects treated with autograft or allograft bone. J Bone Joint Surg Am 2001;83(6):803–16.

18. Seeherman HJ, Azari K, Bidic S, et al. rhBMP-2 delivered in a calcium phosphate cement accelerates bridging of critical-sized defects in rabbit radii. J Bone Joint Surg Am 2006;88(7):1553–65.

19. Aronson J. Limb lengthening, skeletal reconstruction, and bone transport with the Ilizarov method. J Bone Joint Surg Am 1997;79(8):1243–58.

20. Ring D, Allende C, Jafarnia K, et al. United diaphyseal forearm fractures with segmental defects: plate fixation and autogenous cancellous bone grafting. J Bone Joint Surg Am 2004;86(11):2440–5.

21. Ahlmann E, Patzakis M, Roidis N, et al. Comparison of anterior and posterior iliac crest bone grafts in terms of harvest site morbidity and functional outcomes. J Bone Joint Surg Am 2002;84(5):716–20.

22. Seiler JG 3rd, Johnson J. Iliac crest autogenous bone grafting: donor site complications. J South Orthop Assoc 2000;9(2):91–7.

23. Arrington ED, Smith WJ, Chambers HG, et al. Complications of iliac crest bone graft harvesting. Clin Orthop Relat Res 1996;329:300–9.

24. Silber JS, Anderson DG, Daffner SD, et al. Donor site morbidity after anterior iliac crest bone harvest for single-level anterior cervical discectomy and fusion. Spine 2003;28(2):134–9.

25. Masquelet AC. Muscle reconstruction in reconstructive surgery: soft tissue repair and long bone reconstruction. Langenbecks Arch Surg 2003;388(5):344–6.

26. Pelissier P, Masquelet AC, Bareille R, et al. Induced membranes secrete growth factors including vascular and osteoinductive factors and could stimulate bone regeneration. J Orthop Res 2004;22(1):73–9.

27. Hoegel F, Mueller CA, Peter R, et al. Bone debris: dead matter or vital osteoblasts. J Trauma 2004;56(2):363–7.

28. Wenisch S, Trinkaus K, Hild A, et al. Human reaming debris: a source of multipotent stem cells. Bone 2005;36(1):74–83.

29. Frolke JP, Nulend JK, Semeins CM, et al. Viable osteoblastic potential of cortical reamings from intramedullary nailing. J Orthop Res 2004;22(6):1271–5.

30. Schmidmaier G, Herrmann S, Green J, et al. Quantitative assessment of growth factors in reaming aspirate, iliac crest, and platelet preparation. Bone 2006;39(5):1156–63.

31. Polyzois D, Papachristou G, Kotsiopoulos K, et al. Treatment of tibial and femoral bone loss by distraction osteogenesis. Experience in 28 infected and 14 clean cases. Acta Orthop Scand Suppl 1997;275:84–8.

32. Dendrinos GK, Kontos S, Lyritsis E. Use of the Ilizarov technique for treatment of nonunion of the tibia associated with infection. J Bone Joint Surg Am 1995;77(6):835–46.

33. Dagher F, Roukoz S. Compound tibial fractures with bone loss treated by the Ilizarov technique. J Bone Joint Surg Br 1991;73(2):316–21.

34. Masquelet AC, Fitoussi F, Begue T, et al. Reconstruction des os longs par membrane induite et autogreffe spongieuse [Reconstruction of the long bone by the membrane and spongy autograft]. Ann Chir Plast Esthet 2000;45:346–53 [in French].

35. Viateau V, Guillemin G, Calando Y, et al. Induction of a barrier membrane to facilitate reconstruction of massive segmental diaphyseal bone defects: an ovine model. Vet Surg 2006;35:445–52.

36. Zucman J, Maurer P, Berbesson C. Experimental study of osteogenic action of periosteal grafts, bone marrow grafts, and centro-medullary riming. Rev Chir Orthop Reparatrice Appar Mot 1968;54(3):221–38.

37. Chapman MW. Closed intramedullary bone grafting and nailing of segmental defects of the femur. J Bone Joint Surg Am 1980;62(6):1004–8.

38. Tydings JD, Martino LJ, Kircher M, et al. The osteoinductive potential of intramedullary canal bone reamings. Curr Surg 1986;43(2):121–4.

39. Tydings JD, Martino LJ, Kircher M, et al. Viability of intramedullary canal bone reamings for continued calcification. Am J Surg 1987;153(3):306–9.

40. Husebye EE, Lyberg T, Madsen JE, et al. The influence of a one-step reamer-irrigator-aspirator technique on the intramedullary pressure in the pig femur. Injury 2006;37(10):935–40.

41. Higgins TF, Casey V, Bachus K. Cortical heat generation using an irrigating/aspirating single-pass reaming vs conventional stepwise reaming. J Orthop Trauma 2007;21(3):192–7.

42. Pape H, Zelle BA, Hildebrand F, et al. Reamed femoral nailing in sheep: does irrigation and aspiration of intramedullary contents alter the systemic response? J Bone Joint Surg Am 2005;87(11):2515–22.

43. Belthur MV, Conway JD, Jindal G, et al. Bone graft harvest using a new intramedullary system. Clin Orthop Relat Res 2008;466(12):2973–80.

44. Brooker AF, Bowerman JW, Robinson RA, et al. Ectopic ossification following total hip replacement: incidence and a method of classification. J Bone Joint Surg Am 1973;55(8):1629–32.

45. Furlong AJ, Giannoudis PV, Smith RM. Heterotopic ossification: a comparison between reamed and unreamed femoral nailing. Injury 1997;28(1):9–14.

Autograft and Nonunions: Morbidity with Intramedullary Bone Graft versus Iliac Crest Bone Graft

Janet D. Conway, MD

KEYWORDS

- Reamer/Irrigator/Aspirator • Intramedullary • Bone graft
- Nonunion • ICBG • Iliac crest bone graft

Autologous bone graft has always been the gold standard for treating nonunions secondary to the osteoinductive effect of the many bone morphogenetic proteins (BMPs) and the live osteoblasts. Traditionally, autologous bone graft for nonunions has been harvested from the anterior and posterior iliac crest. The iliac crest has many advantages including the availability of large quantities of bone without structural compromise to the extremity. The other advantage of iliac crest bone graft (ICBG), in addition to all the benefits of autologous bone graft, is its ability to be used as a tricortical structural graft. The disadvantages, however, have been well documented in the literature and include persistent donor site pain, numbness surrounding the donor site, infection, and fractures.[1–4]

Recently, a new device, the Reamer/Irrigator/Aspirator (RIA) (Synthes, Inc, West Chester, PA), has been used to harvest autograft from the intramedullary canals of the femur and tibia. Intramedullary bone graft harvest allows for a fairly large volume of bone graft to be harvested when compared with the volume of graft obtained from the iliac crest; however, it also has the advantage of less donor site morbidity. The following article addresses in detail the advantages and disadvantages of obtaining bone graft from the iliac crest versus the intramedullary canals. Specifically, this article will discuss the volume and quality of graft obtained, harvest time, blood loss, postoperative pain, functional impairment, major and minor complications, and the potential for repeat harvesting.

BONE GRAFT VOLUME

Graft volume is a critical consideration when choosing a donor site for autograft. Larger bone graft volumes are needed for segmental defects, and each donor site has a limited supply. Also, regardless of donor site, the bone quality of the patient has a significant impact on the amount of bone graft available with a larger amount of bone available in a young, healthy patient.[5,6] Some studies[1,7] have suggested that when a larger volume of graft is harvested from the anterior or posterior iliac crest, the donor site morbidity increases.

Anterior ICBG volume has been reported to range from an average of 5.3 cm^3 (Bruno and colleagues)[8] to 72 cm^3 (Marx and Morales).[9] Five studies have been published on anterior iliac crest bone graft volume that focus on nonspine usage. Hall and colleagues[10] reported the average volume of compressed cancellous bone was

The author's institution has received a grant from Synthes, Inc (West Chester, PA).
International Center for Limb Lengthening, Rubin Institute for Advanced Orthopedics, Sinai Hospital of Baltimore, 2401 West Belvedere Avenue, Baltimore, MD 21215, USA
E-mail address: jconway@lifebridgehealth.org

Orthop Clin N Am 41 (2010) 75–84
doi:10.1016/j.ocl.2009.07.006

12.87 cm³ (range, 6.6–18.6 cm³) in elderly cadaveric specimens. Kessler and colleagues[2] measured cancellous bone harvested from between the anterior iliac tables and reported an average volume of 9 cm³ (range, 5–12 cm³) with an average patient age of 44 years (range, 8–80 years). Ahlmann and colleagues[1] reported an average volume of 54.3 cm³ (no range reported), but they included the use of the outer cortical table, which was then converted into chips and measured using a medicine cup and syringe. The average age in their study was 46.2 years (range, 12–77 years). The addition of cortical bone graft from the outer table significantly increased the volume obtained. Marx and Morales[9] harvested anterior ICBG for large jaw defects from patients who were 18 to 75 years old. The mean non-compressed volume was 72 cm³.

Posterior ICBG has been traditionally used when larger volumes of bone graft are necessary. Kessler and colleagues[2] reported an average cancellous bone graft volume of 25.5 cm³ (range, 17–29 cm³) from the posterior iliac crest. Kessler and colleagues[2] harvested an average of only 9 cm³ from the anterior iliac crest, which gives the posterior crest a distinct volume advantage. Hall and colleagues[10] reported a similar volume of compressed cancellous bone graft with an average of 30.31 cm³ (range, 27.1–34 cm³). The average posterior ICBG volume in the Ahlmann and colleagues[1] study was 55.12 cm³; however, this also included cortical strips, which significantly increased the available graft volume. Marx and Morales[9] reported an average posterior ICBG harvest of 88 cm³. The posterior ICBG harvest contained significantly more bone than the anterior ICBG harvest (mean, 72 cm³) ($P<.05$).[9]

Belthur and colleagues[5] reported an average intramedullary femoral bone graft volume of 41.1 cm³ (range, 25–75 cm³) with an average patient age of 44.9 years (range, 15–78 years). Scharfenberger and Weber[6] reported an average femoral intramedullary graft volume of 68 cm³ (range, 40–90 cm³) with a much younger average patient age of 34 years (range, 16–53 years). Belthur and colleagues[5] also reported an average tibial graft volume of 32.5 cm³ (range, 25–50 cm³) (**Fig. 1**). Graft volume in femoral and tibial cases is directly dependent on the size of the reamer head chosen for the harvest as well as the patient age. Larger volumes can be harvested with larger reamer heads, but the torsional stability of the canal is compromised if more than the inner 2 mm of cortical bone is resected.[11]

On average, intramedullary bone graft has more graft volume than anterior ICBG and has at least similar bone graft volumes when compared with posterior ICBG (**Table 1**). In the younger population, intramedullary bone graft might provide larger volumes than posterior ICBG.

BONE GRAFT QUALITY

Few studies[12] have compared graft "quality" or the presence of viable cells and growth factors. Frölke and colleagues[12] determined that there are live osteoblasts in cortical reamings of sheep femora. Schmidmaier and colleagues[13] compared the quantity of BMPs in the crest graft versus the intramedullary graft. They reported significantly elevated levels of fibroblast growth factor-alpha (FGFa), platelet-derived growth factor (PDGF), insulin-like growth factor 1 (IGF-1), transforming growth factor beta 1 (TGF-B1), and BMP-2 in the reamings of the intramedullary femoral canal when compared with bone graft from the iliac crest. These studies are encouraging with respect

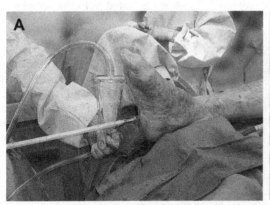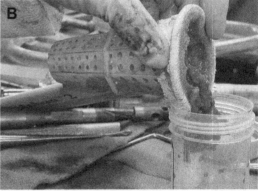

Fig. 1. (*A*), Photograph of an intramedullary graft harvest using the Reamer/Irrigator/Aspirator. This bone graft was used for an ankle and hindfoot fusion using an intramedullary rod. The bone graft was harvested from the intramedullary canal of the tibia. (*B*), Photograph shows one of the many filters used for the intramedullary bone graft harvest. The bone graft is being placed into a measuring cup to determine the quantity of graft harvested and to safely store the graft in the measuring cup with a lid until it is needed.

Table 1
Comparison of bone graft harvest sites: anterior iliac crest, posterior iliac crest, and intramedullary canal

	Anterior Iliac Crest Harvest Site	Posterior Iliac Crest Harvest Site	Intramedullary Canal Harvest Site
Volume of graft obtained	5–72 cm^3	25–88 cm^3	25–90 cm^3
Time to harvest	35 min	40 min + 20 min for repositioning	30 min
Volume of blood loss	Greater than posterior	Less than anterior	Unknown
Acute and chronic pain	Greatest	Intermediate	Least amount of pain
Duration of gait abnormalities	3–4 weeks	2 weeks	1 week
Rate of major complications	Highest rate	Intermediate rate	Lowest rate
Rate of minor complications	Highest rate	Intermediate rate	Lowest rate
Advantages of harvest site	Tricortical support; no repositioning	Tricortical support; good bone graft volume	Large concentration of growth factors; good bone graft volume; minimal complications
Disadvantages of harvest site	Small volume; pain; greatest number of complications	Increased intraoperative time with repositioning	Nonstructural bone graft

to the quality of the intramedullary graft harvested; however, more research is required to see if these advantages are of clinical significance.

HARVEST TIME

Harvest time is a significant factor when choosing an autograft donor site because the bone graft harvest is just one portion of the procedure. Consideration must be given to the location of the recipient site and the additional time necessary for reprepping and draping if the patient needs to be repositioned after the harvest. Kessler and colleagues[2] recorded the average time for harvesting anterior and posterior ICBG. The average anterior iliac crest harvest time was 35 minutes (range, 22–48 minutes), and the average posterior iliac crest harvest time was 40 minutes (range, 32–55 minutes) with an additional average repositioning time of 20 minutes (range, 14–27 minutes).[2] Marx and Morales[9] compared anterior harvest times to posterior harvest times. The average posterior harvest time was 106 minutes versus 134 minutes for the anterior harvest time (P<.08).[9] There was no mention as to whether

repositioning time was included in the posterior harvest.

No formally published studies have recorded the harvest time for the intramedullary femoral graft; however, Belthur and colleagues[14] reported the average intramedullary graft harvest time as 30 minutes (no range reported). The additional advantage of the intramedullary harvest is that even if the contralateral side is harvested, there is no reprepping and repositioning necessary as long as the surgical procedure is performed in the supine position. Nichols and colleagues[15] reported a case of intramedullary bone graft harvest for posterior lumbar fusion in which the intramedullary harvest was performed in the prone position, thus eliminating the need for additional reprepping and draping in these cases.

Intramedullary harvest had the shortest harvest time followed by the anterior iliac crest (see **Table 1**). It is difficult to use the data from the Marx and Morales[9] study because there was no mention of repositioning the patient after the posterior crest harvest. This repositioning would be a necessary part of their procedure because they were using the large posterior graft harvests for large jaw defects.

BLOOD LOSS

Two studies[1,9] have reported the estimated blood loss after ICBG harvest. Ahlmann and colleagues[1] reported the average intraoperative blood loss from posterior ICBG harvest as 75 mL with the total blood loss including the postoperative drain as 169.14 mL. Anterior ICBG harvest intraoperative blood loss was also 75 mL, but when the drain output was added, the total blood loss was 232.47 mL. In this study, the posterior iliac crest harvest had significantly less blood loss ($P \le .018$). Marx and Morales[9] also compared posterior ICBG harvest blood loss with anterior ICBG harvest blood loss. This blood loss estimate included the sponge weights, suction canister volume, and drain output. Posterior crest blood loss averaged 306 mL versus 474 mL for the anterior crest blood loss ($P<.001$).

With respect to intramedullary bone graft harvest, Scharfenberger and Weber[6] used hemoglobin and hematocrit to estimate blood loss after intramedullary harvest in 11 patients. The average hemoglobin drop was 4.3 g/dL (range, 2.3–8.0 g/dL) and the average hematocrit drop was 11% (range, 6%–22%). These data might be altered by the recipient site bleeding and the dilutional effect that the intravenous fluids have on the measurement of hematocrit and hemoglobin. At present, it is difficult to quantify the blood loss after the use of the intramedullary harvesting device and should be the subject of further study.

POSTOPERATIVE PAIN

Multiple studies have documented postoperative pain after anterior and posterior iliac crest graft harvest.[2–4] Many of these studies are in conjunction with spine surgery[16]; however, this section will concentrate on indications other than spine when possible. Donor site pain is underappreciated by the surgeon as shown in a study by Heary and colleagues.[17] Heary and colleagues[17] reported on surgeon perception of persistent donor site pain versus patient perception of persistent donor site pain after spinal surgery. Neurosurgeons appreciated donor site pain only 8% of the time as opposed to the actual incidence of donor site pain reported by patients as 34%.

With respect to acute pain (ie, immediately postoperative or within 1 to 2 months following surgery), a large number of authors report limited activity secondary to pain.[2,4,5] According to DeOrio and Farber[4] who studied pain after harvest from the anterior iliac crest, the acute pain on a 10-point visual analog scale (VAS) averaged 3.8 points (range, 0–10 points) with 108 (84%) of 128 patients

limiting their activity because of pain for 4 weeks or less. Belthur and colleagues[5] also reported acute anterior iliac crest pain using a visual analog scale for frequency and intensity for a maximum total pain score of 20 points. The immediate postoperative pain score obtained at less than 48 hours averaged 12.13 points (range, 9–18 points), and the postoperative pain score obtained less than 3 months after surgery averaged 8.61 (range, 3–15 points). The scores from patients who underwent anterior ICBG harvest were all significantly higher when compared with the intramedullary harvest groups during the same time intervals ($P<.001$).[5] Marx and Morales[9] compared anterior ICBG harvest with posterior ICBG harvest in the acute (day 1 and day 10) postoperative period and showed that the anterior crest donor site was more acutely painful. On postoperative day 1, the mean pain score (on a 10-point VAS) for the anterior harvest was an average of 7.2 ± 1.6 versus an average of 3.1 ± 0.7 for the posterior harvest ($P<.005$). On postoperative day 10, the average score anteriorly was 4.4 ± 0.5 versus an average of 0.3 ± 0.3 posteriorly ($P<.005$).

Most authors also reported some encouraging statistics with respect to resolving acute pain. Three studies[2,4,18] found that 70.0% to 92.2% of acute pain symptoms from anterior ICBG harvest resolved within 4 weeks. DeOrio and Farber[4] reported that 118 of 128 patients had total resolution of their pain at 8 weeks. Weatherby and colleagues[19] reported acute donor site pain following intramedullary graft harvest for nonunion lasting 40 days in only 5 (23%) of 24 patients.

Chronic pain (ie, pain lasting longer than 3 months) is a problem for a small percentage of patients after harvest from the anterior iliac crest. Cricchio and Lundgren[20] reported that 8 (11%) of 70 patients had pain after 2 years and DeOrio and Farber[4] reported that 4 of 128 patients had pain for more than 7 months. Silber and colleagues[16] reported anterior donor site pain after a one-level anterior cervical discectomy and fusion. Thirty-five of 134 patients had chronic pain at the donor site with a mean VAS score of 3.8 points.[16] Fifteen of 134 patients in this study used pain medication for their donor site, and 7 of 134 patients had chronic discomfort with their clothing.[16] Belthur and colleagues[5] also found that chronic pain scores using a VAS for frequency and intensity were significantly higher in the anterior iliac crest group after 3 months with an average of 1.30 points (range, 0–10 points) versus 0.10 points (range, 0–4 points) for the intramedullary harvest group ($P<.001$).

With respect to acute pain following posterior ICBG harvest, Kessler and colleagues[2] reported that 15 (33%) of 46 patients had acute pain that resolved during the following month. No patients in the Kessler and colleagues[2] study experienced chronic pain. Mirovsky and Neuwirth[21] documented postoperative pain using two different methods of posterior iliac crest harvesting. One group (Group A) had bone harvested from the outer table with underlying cancellous bone, and one group (Group B) had cancellous bone harvested from between the tables. Fourteen (56%) of 25 patients in Group A and 12 (52%) of 23 patients in Group B had acute pain during the first week. This number gradually declined during the following 12 months to 6 (24%) of 25 patients in Group A and 4 (17%) of 23 patients in Group B. Chronic pain at 24 months was present in 5 (20%) of 25 patients in Group A and 4 (17%) of 23 patients in Group B.[21]

To summarize the pain data, the anterior iliac crest harvest had more acute pain when compared with posterior iliac crest and intramedullary bone graft harvest (see **Table 1**). No study exists in the literature that compares posterior crest graft with intramedullary graft, so it is difficult to say which one of these sites is less painful. In my opinion, the intramedullary harvest is ultimately less painful secondary to the very small (1–2 cm) incision required for harvest and the ability to harvest bone without any muscle dissection off of the bone as in the posterior crest harvest. It is interesting to note that in the Belthur and colleagues[5] study, six patients underwent anterior ICBG harvest and intramedullary harvest at two different points in time. All six patients said that the intramedullary graft harvest was much less painful in all time periods when compared with their previous anterior ICBG harvest.[5] With respect to the chronic pain data, intramedullary donor site has the least amount of chronic pain followed by the posterior iliac crest and then anterior iliac crest.

GAIT ABNORMALITIES AND FUNCTIONAL IMPAIRMENT

Many studies have documented gait disturbances after anterior ICBG harvest. Several authors[2,4,18,20] reported acute gait disturbances within the first 2 to 4 weeks that resulted in patients having a limp or using crutches. Most of these gait disturbances resolved after 1 month; however, Marx and Morales[9] reported that 8 (15%) of 50 of patients still had a limp at postoperative day 60 secondary to the anterior ICBG harvest. DeOrio and Farber[4] also reported that 2 (1.5%) of 129 patients had persistent walking difficulty because of the graft site and

Cricchio and Lundgren[20] reported 3 patients with gait problems 2 years after harvest.

Silber and colleagues[16] documented chronic functional impairment after anterior ICBG harvest for a one-level anterior discectomy and fusion. Some patients (12.7%) had difficulty with ambulation and 11.9% were limited in their recreational activities secondary to donor site pain.[16] Fewer than 10% of the patients in this study reported difficulty with activities of daily living, limited ability to complete household chores, restricted work activities, and restricted sexual activities.[16]

Gait disturbances after posterior ICBG harvest were documented by Kessler and colleagues[2] with 3 (6%) of 46 patients having gait abnormalities at 2 weeks and only 1 person with persistent gait problems at 4 weeks. Marx and Morales[9] reported that the average first day of ambulation after posterior ICBG harvest was 1.7 days. This was significantly better than the anterior ICBG harvest group who had mean first day of ambulation of 3.6 days (P<.005).[9] The number of patients limping on postoperative day 10 (6% versus 42%) and postoperative day 60 (0% versus 15%) was significantly fewer in the posterior ICBG group than the anterior ICBG group (P<.005).[9]

Gait disturbances with intramedullary bone graft harvest were documented by Belthur and colleagues[14] and compared with anterior ICBG harvest. Patients who underwent intramedullary bone graft harvest had an average time for ambulatory dysfunction of 1 week versus patients who underwent anterior ICBG harvest who had an average time of 3 weeks for ambulatory dysfunction. Given these data, the intramedullary bone harvest has the least impact on ambulation postoperatively, followed by posterior ICBG harvest and then anterior ICBG harvest (see **Table 1**).

MAJOR COMPLICATIONS

According to Younger and Chapman,[3] major complications are complications that require surgical intervention, require additional days in the hospital, or cause significant permanent sequelae or disability. Multiple studies[1,3,5,9,20] have documented major complications after anterior ICBG harvest. Ahlmann and colleagues[1] documented persistent lateral femoral cutaneous nerve numbness in five (8%) patients and one abdominal hernia. Cricchio and Lundgren[20] reported one iliac wing fracture treated nonoperatively and two neurologic injuries to the lateral femoral cutaneous nerve. **Fig. 2** shows an example of a symptomatic iliac wing fracture with a large abdominal hernia. In the study of Belthur and colleagues,[5] 40 patients underwent anterior ICBG harvest. Four patients

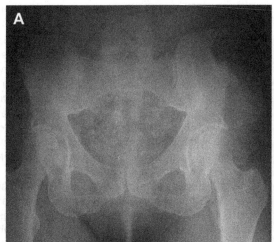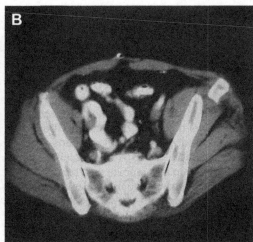

Fig. 2. (*A*), Anteroposterior view radiograph of a devastating complication after anterior iliac crest graft harvest for an anterior spinal fusion. The radiograph shows a large fracture of the anterior superior iliac spine with displacement. (*B*), Image of the same patient obtained using computed tomography shows the herniation of abdominal contents into the fracture gap. The fracture and hernia were surgically repaired by a team of orthopedic and general surgeons.

(10%) had major complications (three deep infections and one hematoma requiring surgical intervention). Marx and Morales[9] reported 50 cases of anterior ICBG harvest for massive jaw reconstruction. They had a 12% incidence of seroma and 6% incidence of hematoma. They also reported a stress fracture of the anterior ilium requiring prolonged rest and activity limitation for 2 months.

Younger and Chapman[3] reported one of the largest series of patients with ICBG harvest. They divided the anterior ICBG harvests into two groups: those with harvest from the outer iliac table and those with harvest from the inner table. The complication rate from the outer table was 3.1% (65 patients), and the complication rate from the inner table harvest was 18.2% (11 patients).[3] Their reported complications included severe pain, nerve injury, osteomyelitis, reoperation for deep infection, prolonged wound drainage, and large hematoma. Younger and Chapman[3] attributed the higher complication rate with the inner table harvest to the potential for increased traction on the lateral femoral cutaneous nerve as well as additional dissection. Careful placement of the incision (**Fig. 3**A) can help to avoid this complication. Also of note in this study[3] was the large number of patients (84 of 239 patients) with significant medical comorbidities. The major complication rate in these patients was significantly higher (14.3%) than in those who did not have preexisting medical illnesses (5.8%) (*P* = .02).[3]

Major complications from posterior ICBG harvest include hematomas, residual numbness, deep infection, and vascular injuries. Arrington and colleagues[22] reported three cases of superior gluteal arterial injuries requiring surgical treatment. Ahlmann and colleagues[1] reported a major complication rate of 2% (one of 42 patients); the one patient had numbness lasting more than 6 months at the donor site as a result of damage to the cluneal nerves. Kessler and colleagues[2] reported seromas in 3 of 46 patients and hematomas in 2 of 46 patients. The study of Marx and Morales[9] had 50 patients who had posterior ICBG harvested; 1 patient developed a seroma that was treated nonoperatively. Younger and Chapman[3] reported 87 posterior ICBG harvest sites with a major complication rate of 5.7%. These complications included osteomyelitis and long-term sensory loss. See **Fig. 3**B for ideal posterior incision placement.

Forty intramedullary graft harvests were reported by Belthur and colleagues,[5] and one major complication was observed. This complication was secondary to an aggressive pyriformis start and a large-diameter reamer head, which resulted in a potential stress riser in the femoral neck. The ideal placement of the incision for the intramedullary harvest of the femur is shown in **Fig. 3**C. Images were obtained postoperatively using computed tomography, and they showed a large channel in the femoral neck. Based on this information, the surgeon elected to prophylactically insert cannulated screws into the femoral neck for stabilization. Belthur and colleagues[5] do not report any long-term major complications. There were no incidences of paresthesia or infections. Scharfenberger and Weber[6] reported on their experience with 11 patients using intramedullary graft harvest for segmental bone defects. They reported

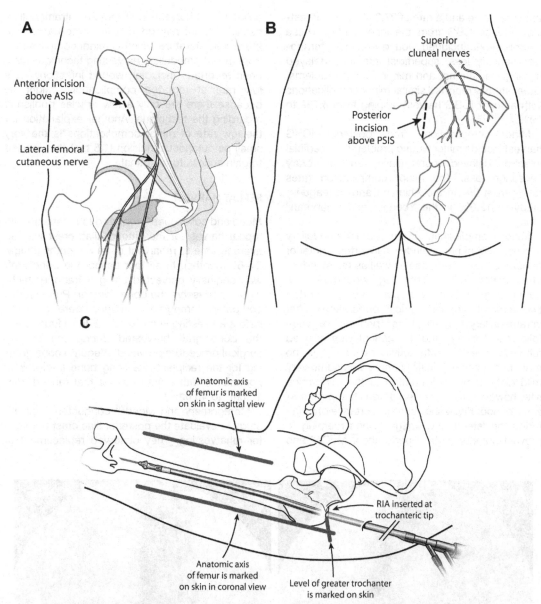

Fig. 3. (*A*), Illustration shows the ideal placement of the incision for anterior iliac crest bone graft harvest to avoid damage to the lateral femoral cutaneous nerve. *ASIS*, anterior superior iliac spine. (*B*), Illustration shows the ideal placement of the incision for posterior iliac crest bone graft harvest to avoid damage to the cluneal nerves. *PSIS*, posterior superior iliac spine. (*C*), Illustration shows the placement of the incision to allow the Reamer/Irrigator/ Aspirator (*RIA*) system to harvest intramedullary bone graft from the femur.

a postoperative bleed as their one donor site complication. It was not specified whether this bleed required operative intervention. Weatherby and colleagues[19] reported 24 cases of intramedullary graft harvest for nonunion without any major complications.

To summarize the major complication rate, the intramedullary harvest has the lowest morbidity followed by the posterior ICBG harvest (see **Table 1**). The anterior ICBG harvest had the largest

number of major complications in numerous studies.[1,3,5,9,20]

MINOR COMPLICATIONS

Minor complications, according to Younger and Chapman,[3] are those that do not cause permanent impairment and resolve with minimal treatment. They reported a minor complication rate of 24.6% for anterior ICBG when harvesting from the outer table and a rate of 27.3% when harvesting anterior ICBG from the inner table.[3] These complications included wound drainage, temporary sensory loss, superficial infection, delayed healing, hematoma, and minor wound problems. Other studies reported similar minor complications with anterior ICBG harvest ranging from 4.7% to 29%.[1–5,16,18]

Minor complications from posterior ICBG harvest include minor wound problems, superficial infection, delayed wound healing, and temporary sensation loss. The minor complication rates range from 0% in the Ahlmann and colleagues[1] study to 12.6% in the Younger and Chapman[3] study.

Minor complications from the intramedullary harvest technique include inadvertent anterior femoral cortex perforation as well as the standard other minor complications (eg, wound healing, hematoma). Belthur and colleagues[5] reported two femoral anterior cortical perforations after intramedullary harvest. These perforations were followed clinically, and the patient was allowed full weight bearing with activity restriction (ie, no running or jumping). Initially, there was some very mild distal femoral discomfort at the perforation site; however, this resolved gradually during a 4-week period. **Fig. 4** shows the importance of monitoring the lateral view images when reaming to prevent anterior cortical perforation. McCall and colleagues[23] harvested 21 femoral intramedullary canals without any donor site complications. In the current literature, no other minor complications from the intramedullary harvesting technique have been reported—including wound infections. This low rate of reported complications might be because there are only a few articles published regarding the technique. Another explanation for the low rate of minor complications is the very small percutaneous incision (1.5 cm) that is used to gain access to the canal.

REPEAT HARVEST

Moed and colleagues[24] reported four patients with repeat harvest of the anterior iliac crest with an average time to reharvest of 34.5 months (range, 24–60 months). In all four cases, the bone graft was originally harvested using a trapdoor technique to preserve the bone contour. Preoperative computed tomography images were obtained before harvesting in these cases. In all four cases, the bone graft harvested during the second surgical procedure provided adequate bone grafting for the recipient site (long bone fractures or nonunions) with a graft volume that ranged from 15 cm^3 to 40 cm^3.[24]

Montgomery and Moed[25] conducted a canine study to evaluate the posterior iliac crest potential for reharvesting. They observed replacement of

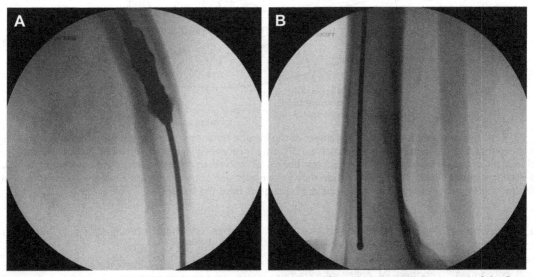

Fig. 4. (*A*), Lateral view radiograph shows bone graft being harvested from the intramedullary canal of the femur. Note how important it is to check the lateral view radiograph. The femur shown has a very large anterior bow, which puts the anterior cortex in jeopardy with any additional reaming. Note the lucency near the tip of the reamer where the anterior cortex was starting to be reamed away. (*B*), Lateral view radiograph shows a more ideal position of the guide wire for the intramedullary reaming of the femur. However, note the close proximity of the anterior cortex to the guide wire. Great care must be taken with reaming by checking the lateral view radiograph frequently to ensure that there are no anterior cortical violations.

new cancellous bone after 1 year based on radiographic and histologic analysis. Fracture healing models have suggested that canines have double the healing rate as humans.[25,26] Montgomery and Moed[25] suggest that reharvest of the posterior iliac crest might be possible in humans after 2 years.

In my personal experience, three patients required repeat femoral harvesting for bone grafting. Two patients required bone grafting of different sites than the original recipient site, and the third patient required bone grafting of the same recipient nonunion site. These repeat harvests were performed between 0.75 years and 3.00 years after the original harvest. The bone graft volumes obtained during the repeat harvest were 35 cm^3, 50 cm^3, and 65 cm^3. No additional donor site complications occurred after the repeat harvest. In the case that required repeat harvest at 9 months, more bone graft was harvested during the second harvest than the initial harvest. This increase in volume can potentially be attributed to the fracture response and remodeling that occurs after reaming. This did not appear to occur in the remaining two harvests as the time period between harvests was longer and the bone might have had more time to remodel to normal density.

SUMMARY

The intramedullary graft has the least patient morbidity at the donor site for nonunions. It is harvested through a nearly percutaneous incision with the potential for repeat harvests. Very few clinical papers are published about intramedullary bone grafts. As more surgeons embrace this technique, there might be more reports that show an increase in patient donor site morbidity. However, in my experience of nearly 100 intramedullary graft harvests, I have been extremely satisfied with the quality, quantity, and minimal morbidity of intramedullary bone graft. The author almost exclusively uses intramedullary graft. One of the only drawbacks of the intramedullary harvest is the inability to provide structural support in the shape of a tricortical graft. It is not often that a tricortical graft would be needed in a nonunion unless a segmental defect was present. When a nonunion would require a tricortical segment, the site with the least donor site morbidity is the posterior iliac crest. The reduced blood loss and fewer number of complications, however, are a trade-off that the surgeon must critically assess in light of the increase in operative time associated with repositioning.

ACKNOWLEDGMENTS

I thank Amanda Chase, MA, for her editing expertise; Joy Marlowe, MA, for her excellent illustrations; and Alvien Lee for his assistance in preparing the figures for publication.

REFERENCES

1. Ahlmann E, Patzakis M, Roidis N, et al. Comparison of anterior and posterior iliac crest bone grafts in terms of harvest-site morbidity and functional outcomes. J Bone Joint Surg Am 2002; 84(5):716–20.
2. Kessler P, Thorwarth M, Bloch-Birkholz A, et al. Harvesting of bone from the iliac crest—comparison of the anterior and posterior sites. Br J Oral Maxillofac Surg 2005;43(1):51–6.
3. Younger EM, Chapman MW. Morbidity at bone graft donor sites. J Orthop Trauma 1989;3(3):192–5.
4. DeOrio JK, Farber DC. Morbidity associated with anterior iliac crest bone grafting in foot and ankle surgery. Foot Ankle Int 2005;26(2):147–51.
5. Belthur MV, Conway JD, Jindal G, et al. Bone graft harvest using a new intramedullary system. Clin Orthop Relat Res 2008;466(12):2973–80.
6. Scharfenberger AV, Weber TG. Reamer irrigation aspirator (RIA) for bone graft harvest: applications for grafting large segmental defects in the tibia and femur. Poster presented at: Orthopaedic Trauma Association Annual Meeting; October 20–22, 2005; Ottawa, Ontario.
7. Kurz LT, Garfin SR, Booth RE Jr. Harvesting autogenous iliac bone grafts. A review of complications and techniques. Spine 1989;14(12):1324–31.
8. Bruno RJ, Cohen MS, Berzins A, et al. Bone graft harvesting from the distal radius, olecranon, and iliac crest: a quantitative analysis. J Hand Surg Am 2001;26(1):135–41.
9. Marx RE, Morales MJ. Morbidity from bone harvest in major jaw reconstruction: a randomized trial comparing the lateral anterior and posterior approaches to the ilium. J Oral Maxillofac Surg 1988;46(3):196–203.
10. Hall MB, Vallerand WP, Thompson D, et al. Comparative anatomic study of anterior and posterior iliac crests as donor sites. J Oral Maxillofac Surg 1991; 49(6):560–3.
11. Pratt DJ, Papagiannnopoulos G, Rees PH, et al. The effects of medullary reaming on the torsional strength of the femur. Injury 1987;18:177–9.
12. Frölke JP, Nulend JK, Semeins CM, et al. Viable osteoblastic potential of cortical reamings from intramedullary nailing. J Orthop Res 2004;22(6):1271–5.
13. Schmidmaier G, Herrmann S, Green J, et al. Quantitative assessment of growth factors in reaming

aspirate, iliac crest, and platelet preparation. Bone 2006;39(5):1156–63.

14. Belthur MV, Conway JD, Ranade A, et al. Use of the reamer/irrigator/aspirator (RIA) to harvest bone graft for limb reconstruction surgery: technique, early experience, and outcomes. Paper presented at: The Limb Lengthening and Reconstruction Society 17th Annual Meeting. Chicago (IL), July 20–22, 2007.

15. Nichols TA, Sagi HC, Weber TG, et al. An alternative source of autograft bone for spinal fusion: the femur: technical case report. Neurosurgery 2008;62(3 Suppl 1):E179 [discussion: E179].

16. Silber JS, Anderson DG, Daffner SD, et al. Donor site morbidity after anterior iliac crest bone harvest for single-level anterior cervical discectomy and fusion. Spine 2003;28(2):134–9.

17. Heary RF, Schlenk RP, Sacchieri TA, et al. Persistent iliac crest donor site pain: independent outcome assessment. Neurosurgery 2002;50(3):510–6 [discussion: 516–7].

18. Rawashdeh MA. Morbidity of iliac crest donor site following open bone harvesting in cleft lip and palate patients. Int J Oral Maxillofac Surg 2008; 37(3):223–7.

19. Weatherby B, Rudd J, Norris BL, et al. Reamer irrigator aspirator (RIA) bone graft harvesting in nonunion and segmental defect repair. Poster presented at: American Academy of Orthopaedic Surgeons Annual Meeting. San Diego (CA), February 14–18, 2007.

20. Cricchio G, Lundgren S. Donor site morbidity in two different approaches to anterior iliac crest bone harvesting. Clin Implant Dent Relat Res 2003;5(3):161–9.

21. Mirovsky Y, Neuwirth MG. Comparison between the outer table and intracortical methods of obtaining autogenous bone graft from the iliac crest. Spine 2000;25(13):1722–5.

22. Arrington ED, Smith WJ, Chambers HG, et al. Complications of iliac crest bone graft harvesting. Clin Orthop Relat Res 1996;(329):300–9.

23. McCall T, Weber T, Brokaw D, et al. Treatment of large segmental bone defects with reamer-irrigator-aspirator bone graft. Paper presented at: Orthopaedic Trauma Association Annual Meeting. Boston, (MA), October 17–20, 2007.

24. Moed BR, Thorderson N, Linden MD. Reharvest of iliac crest donor site cancellous bone. Clin Orthop Relat Res 1998;(346):223–7.

25. Montgomery DM, Moed BR. Cancellous bone donor site regeneration. J Orthop Trauma 1989;3(4):290–4.

26. Schenk R, Willenegger H. Morphological findings in primary fracture healing. Symp Biol Hung 1967;7:75–86.

Autologous Bone Graft: When Shall We Add Growth Factors?

Peter V. Giannoudis, BSc, MB, MD, FRCS[a,b],*,
Haralampos T. Dinopoulos, MD[a]

KEYWORDS
• Nonunion • Bone defect • Autologous bone graft
• Growth factors • Graft expansion • BMPs

Despite the ongoing advances in the treatment of fractures and understanding of the fracture repair processes, impaired healing continues to be one of the most debilitating complications of fractures. Up to 10% of the 6.2 million fractures occurring annually in the United States are associated with impaired healing.[1] Many of these cases of impaired fracture healing demonstrate unique characteristics posed not only by the initial trauma sustained with bone defects and impaired vascularity of the area but also as a result of previous treatment modalities. Many of these patients require lengthy treatments associated with both functional and psychosocial impairment. Not less worthy is the economical burden to the patient and the health system.[2]

The standard treatment of most aseptic nonunions is mechanical stabilization with or without biologic stimulation depending on the assessment and classification of the nonunion.[3]

The current gold standard for any given situation requiring bone grafting and especially in situations of fracture nonunion is autologous bone grafting (ABG). Autologous cancellous bone grafting remains a unique biologic method promoting union by stimulating the local biology at the nonunion site.[4–7] Autologous bone has all three components necessary to promote or enhance bone regeneration: an osteoconductive scaffold, endogenous bioactive molecules, and cells that are able to respond to these signals. Unfortunately, although autogenous bone is considered as the best graft option, significant complications have been reported related to the harvesting site, most often being the anterior iliac crest of the pelvis.[8] Furthermore, the desirable quantity of the required graft at times may be insufficient.[8]

For these reasons, over the years other biologically based strategies have been developed. These include electrical, ultrasound, and shockwave stimulation, a wide range of bone graft substitutes with either osteoconductive or both osteoconductive and osteoinductive properties, and biologic response modifiers that are administered either locally or systemically, including bone morphogenetic proteins (BMPs), platelet-derived growth factors, and parathyroid hormone.[9–11] These biologic response modifiers, appear to have been used successfully in managing nonunions.[12–14] In addition to nonunion, the administration of these molecules has been used in many other orthopedic situations, including stabilization of implants,[15,16] restoration of large segmental bone defects,[15,17] treatment of osteonecrosis of the femoral head,[18] fusion of joints, cartilage regeneration,[19,20] augmentation of periprosthetic fractures, and acceleration of fracture healing, especially in patients at high risk of fracture nonunion.[21]

[a] Department of Trauma & Orthopedic Surgery, University of Leeds, Leeds General Infirmary, Great George Street, Leeds LS1 3EX, UK
[b] Academic Trauma & Orthopedic Unit, Floor A Clarendon Wing, Leeds General Infirmary University Hospital, Great George Street, Leeds LS1 3EX, UK
* Corresponding author. Academic Trauma & Orthopedic Unit, Floor A Clarendon Wing, Leeds General Infirmary University Hospital, Great George Street, Leeds LS1 3EX.
E-mail address: pgiannoudi@aol.com (P.V. Giannoudis).

Orthop Clin N Am 41 (2010) 85–94
doi:10.1016/j.ocl.2009.07.004
0030-5898/09/$ – see front matter © 2010 Elsevier Inc. All rights reserved.

Nonetheless, there are still adverse clinical settings where despite providing the best mechanical environment modification complemented with ABG, failure has occurred.[22–27] In addition, there are circumstances where the application of growth factors in isolation would not seem enough to promote successful bone healing.[28]

In this study, therefore, we consider in what clinical situations implantation of autologous bone grafting may need enhancement with commercially available growth factors (BMP-2 and BMP-7) to promote successful bone healing.

THE USE OF AUTOLOGOUS BONE GRAFTING OR REAMING BY-PRODUCTS

Tibia is the most common long bone to sustain a fracture. It has a high risk of developing nonunion because of the compromised soft tissue envelope especially over its anterior medial area.[25,29] Consequently, it represents the bone with the highest overall incidence of nonunion, and the "nonunion model."[25]

In the atrophic nonunions, the biologic factor is considered to be mostly the problem, despite the perception that the vascularity at the nonunion site is not compromised. The oligotrophic and even more the atrophic nonunions present insufficient blood supply, or insufficient quantities of bone-forming cells. As a result, augmentation of this poor biologic environment through graft expansion is considered mandatory in achieving union in these difficult nonunion cases.[27,30–34] Several reports exist in the literature illustrating the efficacy of autologous iliac crest bone graft (AICBG) in isolation but also in combination with other materials. Overall the success rate with AIGBG is approximately 80% to 90%.[35–42]

The biologic properties of the "by-products" of reaming (RBP) have gained special interest very early in the history of reamed intramedullary nailing (IMN), representing an internal autografting procedure during closed reamed nailing.[17,43–45] IMN and reaming offers the unique biomechanical advantages of an intramedullary splinting fixation, in association with the osteoinductive stimulus of the "by-products" of reaming.[23,44–46] The vascular flow between endosteum and periosteum of the long bones retains nutrition and healing of the nonunion sites even after the temporary destruction of the endosteal blood flow until it is restored.[47] Although it is debatable in the literature whether to perform the IMN procedure openly or closed, it seems that surgeons open the nonunion site in those cases where the existing hardware needs to be removed, in cases with severe malalignment, and in those cases where additional bone graft needs to be added owing to massive bony defects.[43,48–53] Reckling and Waters[54] reported favorable results in the series of 33 noninfected tibial nonunions that were treated with a posterolateral approach and cortico-cancellous bone application. On an average of 5 months solid healing was noted in 94% of the patients.

Megas and colleagues[53] treated 50 cases of aseptic tibial nonunions with reamed interlocking nail. On average the reamed IMN was performed 15.6 months post injury. Various primary fixation methods were used and 36% had been open fractures. A closed IMN was attempted in all cases, but in 16 an open procedure was finally performed because of irreducible malalignment or for removal of previous hardware. Autologous cancellous graft was added in three cases because of the extent of the bone deficit. All fractures united in a 6-month period post nailing and the method was advocated as highly effective and safe for aseptic tibial nonunions.

In 1999, Wu and colleagues[55] evaluated 25 cases of tibia shaft aseptic nonunions treated with exchange nailing. Most (88.9%) of the original fractures were closed, stabilized with dynamic nails and developed atrophic nonunions. Exchange nailing was performed without opening the nonunion site and the success rates were significant (96%) in an average period of 16 weeks.

In 2003, Wu presented another series[56] of treating tibial aseptic nonunions with reamed IMN. In this study the original fixation method was plating and in 28 cases with adequate follow-up progressed to union. On average, the nonunions healed in 4.5 months (3.0–7.5) after removal of the original plate fixation, excessive reaming of the medullary canal, and insertion of a Kuntscher nail (13 cases) or locked gerhard küntscher (GK) nail (15 cases). However, the author suggested that whenever a large bony defect is present there should be additional bone grafting from the iliac crest and not performing excessive reaming of the medullary canal.

In the series of Devnani,[24] long-bone fracture nonunions were treated with compression plate fixation and AICBG. Among them the author evaluated the time to union of 10 tibial aseptic nonunions, 8 atrophic and 2 hypertrophic. All of the tibial nonunions of this series united at an average of 19.8 weeks, with a satisfactory functional outcome.

A comparative study of Johnson and Marder for tibial aseptic nonunions treated with IMN was published in 1987.[50] The authors used open IMN techniques and compared the effect on healing rates of bone grafting the nonunion site with the by-products of reaming, or with AICBG. Eleven atrophic and 11 hypertrophic cases were evaluated. Successfully treated were 20 nonunion sites (91.9%), with an average time to union of 12.5 weeks. A statistically significant difference between the atrophic and hypertrophic cases (14.4 vs 10.6 weeks, respectively) was identified. The authors compared their results with those of closed IMN techniques and identified major differences in the time to union in favor of their own open nailing techniques.

Sledge and colleagues[51] have described their experience with static reamed IMN for a period of 6 years. Forty aseptic tibial nonunions were treated with reamed arbeitsgemeinschaft für osteosynthesefragen (AO) or GK nails. The original injury in 18 of them was an open fracture and opening of the fracture site was used in 27 (67.5%) of them for removal of implants, proper realignment, and also for AICBG enhancement. The average time to union was 7.1 months (12–67) and the union rates were 100%. No statistically significant differences were observed between open or closed IMN techniques and the use or not of AICBG for enhancement.

An overview of articles with the proven value of AICBG and RBPs is presented in **Table 1**.

THE USE OF GROWTH FACTORS

Aiming to overcome the limitations of the autologous bone grafting, bone morphogenetic proteins (BMP-7 and BMP-2) were produced by recombinant DNA technology.[57,58] They are substances with great osteoinductive properties for the enhancement of bone regeneration in various clinical applications, including the treatment of fracture nonunions.[8,59,60] The safety of their administration, combined with the lack of morbidity and the quantity restrictions that characterize autologous bone grafts, have given to this family of molecules a principal role over the other bone graft substitutes.[22]

The initial experimental in vivo and vitro work on BMPs opened the way for the study of Friedlaender and colleagues that started in 1992 and published in 2001.[12] In their milestone work, they evaluated the application of rhBMP-7 (recombinant human bone morphogenic protein-7 or OP1) in tibial nonunions. One hundred and twenty-four tibia aseptic nonunions were enrolled in a multicenter randomized prospective controlled trial. Either rhBMP-7 (in 63 nonunions) or autologous bone graft (in 61 nonunions) was used for enhancement of nonunion healing. The method of fixation was IMN for all cases (locked in 92%). At 9 months postsurgery, 62% of the rhBMP-7 group and 74% of the AICBG group demonstrated

radiological union ($P = .158$). Overall, the rhBMP-7 administration was safe and proved to be statistically comparable to the gold standard biologic enhancement of autograft. This randomized trial of Friedlaender and colleagues[12] has established BMPs as a bone graft option (see **Table 1**).

The work of Cook[61] (animal model) showed the efficacy of recombinant human osteogenic protein-1 in healing 2-cm segmental defects in nonhuman primates (in ulnae and tibia), whereas the controls filled with AICBG showed only little new bone formation.

This ability of BMPs to regenerate new bone was used in various situations. Following the work of Friedlaender and colleagues the tibia per se is the first model for clinical investigation of potential application of the BMPs.[12] They have been associated with augmenting standard fixation and grafting methods in the acute setting of fractures as well as in established nonunions.[12,21]

Lately, the use of BMPs enhanced with autologous grafting is emerging in literature in various adverse scenarios (**Table 2**).

In a multicenter registry and database (six university centers) observational study, Kanakaris and colleagues[62] focused on the application of BMP-7/OP-1. They presented the preliminary results, of a prospective case series of aseptic tibial nonunions. Sixty-eight patients fulfilled the inclusion criteria for this observational study, with a minimum follow-up of 12 months. The median duration of tibial nonunion before BMP-7 application was 23 months (range 9–317). Patients had undergone a median of 2 (0–11) revision procedures before the administration of BMP-7. In 41%, the application of BMP-7 was combined with revision of the fixation at the nonunion site. In 25 cases (36.8%), the BMP-7 was expanded with the use of autologous bone graft (AICBG), out of which 14 (56%) had been previously treated unsuccessfully with ABG. Nonunion healing was verified in 61 (89.7%) of 68 in a median period of 6.5 months (range 3–15).

Ronga and colleagues,[63] in an observational, retrospective, nonrandomized study on the use of BMP-7, reported on treating nonunions in various anatomic sites. The work was performed by the BMP-7 Italian Observational Study (BIOS) Group. The clinical series included 105 patients. Additional grafts were used based on the surgeon's decision. Radiographic and clinical assessments were performed at progressive time intervals on two groups: BMP-7 + autograft (A) or BMP-7 alone (B). The mean follow-up was 29.2 months. The last assessment showed an overall 88.8% success rate with an average healing time of 7.9 months. In complicated cases, the

Table 1
Articles referring to union rates of fractures enhanced either with iliac crest autologous graft or with reamed–by products

Author Year	Anatomic Site	Method	Graft Used	Results/Union Rates
Reckling & Waters 1980[54]	Tibial 11 closed # 22 open #	Plaster	33 ICAG	93.9%
Johnson & Marder 1987[50]	tibial treatment nonunion fractures	22 tibial # 8 closed # 11 open # (All open # IMN)	10 ICAG 12 RBP	90.9%
Sledge et al 1989[51]	40 tibial #s 18 closed # 22 open #	13 AO nails 27 GK nails 13 closed 27 open	10 ICAG 40 RBP	100%
Wiss et al 1992[30]	50 tibial #s 4 closed 46 open	All compression plating	39 ICAG	96%
Wiss & Stetson 1994[23]	47 tibial #s 14 closed 33 open	IMN	47 RBP	89%
Wu et al 1999[55]	25 closed #s	Reamed IMN	25 RBP	96%
Devnani 2001[24]	10 tibial #s 3 closed 7 open	All compression plating	10 ICAG	100%
Friedlaender et al 2001[12]	124 tibial #s 53 closed 71 open	Locked IMN	61 ICAG 63 BMP-7	62% versus 74%
Megas et al 2001[53]	50 tibial #s 32 closed # 18 open #	GK reamed IMN 34 closed technique 16 open	50 RBP 3 ICAG	100%
Wu 2003[56]	28 tibial #s 25 closed # 3 open #	13 GK 15 Kuntscher all open	28 RBP	100%

Abbreviations: BMP, bone morphogenetic protein; ICAG, iliac crest autologous graft; IMN, intramedullary nailing; RBP, reamed by-products.

success of the BMP-7 + autograft group reached 83.3% compared with 76.5% of the standalone BMP-7. If fewer than three operations preceded, healing was 90.6% compared with 87.8% (BMP-7), and if more than 3 operations preceded, the success dropped to 77.8% compared with 75.0% of BMP-7. At 9 months there was overlapping between the unions recorded in the two groups with healing rates of 86.0% and 85.7%, respectively. This is an observational study that illustrates the efficacy of BMP-7 with and without bone grafting for the treatment of long bone nonunions. This type of observation is confirmed by the comparison of the results between the BMP-7 alone group and

the BMP-7 + autograft group. The increase in the percentage rate of consolidations at different follow-up shows that the interval between 6 and 9 months is a period that can still be considered useful before declaring failure of the treatment. The overlapping of the results according to the variables "previous complications and number of previous operations" confirms the efficacy of BMP-7.

Dimitriou and colleagues[64] in their recent study evaluated the efficacy and safety of recombinant bone morphogenetic protein-7 (rhBMP-7 or OP-1) as a bone-stimulating agent in the treatment of persistent fracture nonunions. Twenty-five patients with 26 fracture nonunions were treated

Table 2
Articles referring to union rates of fractures enhanced with growth factors

Authors	Anatomic Site	Graft Used	Results	Comments
Vaccaro et al 2003[28]	Posterolateral lumbar fusions - No instrumentation	rhBMP-7 (OP-1) + ICAG	- 6/11 pts (55%) with radiographic solid fusion (study criteria) - 10/11 pts (91%) bridging bone on the AP film	Pilot safety and efficacy study of rhBMP-7 (OP-1)
Dimitriou et al 2005[64]	26 persistent upper and lower limb atrophic nonunions	- 17 (65.4%) ABG + rhBMP-7, - 1 (3.8%) case Freeze Dried Allograft + rhBMP-7	- 16/17 (94.1%) clinical & radiological union. - only rhBMP-7 8/9 (88.9%) union	Persistent long-bone atrophic nonunions
Ronga et al 2006[63]	105 patients - 69 lower limp - 36 upper limp	38 only BMP-7 - 11 with an osteoconductive - 50 with ABG - 6 composite graft	90.6% (<2 operations) 77.8% (>3 operations)	Observational, retrospective, nonrandomized (BMP-7 Italian Observational Study [BIOS] Group)
Kanakaris et al 2008[62]	68 tibial aseptic nonunions 41% revision of the fixation 26 (38.2%) ORIF; 7 (10.3%) IMN; 6 (8.8%) Ex Fix	BMP-7/OP-1 in all Graft expansion with autograft 25, 36.8%	61 (89.7%)	multicenter registry and database (6 University centers) observational study

Abbreviations: ABG, autologous cancellous bone graft; AP, anteroposterior; BMP, bone morphogenetic protein; Ex-Fix, external fixator; ICAG, iliac crest autologous graft; IMN, intramedullary nailing; ORIF, open reduction internal fixation; rhBMP-7, recombinant human bone morphogenic protein-7 or OP1.

with rhBMP-7. There were 10 tibial nonunions, 8 femoral, 3 humeral, 3 ulnar, 1 patellar, and 1 clavicular nonunion. The mean follow-up was 15.3 months. The mean number of operations performed before rhBMP-7 application was 3.2, with autologous bone graft and bone marrow injection being used in 10 cases (38.5%). Both clinical and radiological union occurred in 24 (92.3%) cases, within a mean time of 4.2 months and 5.6 months, respectively. No complications or adverse effects from the use of rhBMP-7 were encountered. In 17 (65.4%) cases the BMP application was combined with AICBG. In 16 of these 17 cases nonunion healing was noted. From those who had only rhBMP-7 applied, 8 of 9 healed. Their study supports the view of application of rhBMP-7 combined with autologous bone grafting for the treatment of persistent fracture nonunions.

Vaccaro and colleagues[28] in a pilot safety and efficacy study examined rhBMP-7 (OP-1) as an adjunct to iliac crest autograft in posterolateral lumbar fusions. They combined OP-1 putty with autograft for intertransverse process fusion of the lumbar spine in patients with symptomatic spinal stenosis and degenerative spondylolisthesis following spinal decompression. Twelve patients underwent laminectomy and partial or complete medial facetectomy as required for decompression of the neural elements followed by intertransverse process fusion by placing iliac crest autograft and OP-1 putty between the decorticated transverse processes. No instrumentation was used. Patients were followed clinically using the Oswestry scale and radiographically using static and dynamic radiographs to assess their fusion status. Radiographic outcome was compared with a historical control (autograft alone fusion without instrumentation for the treatment of degenerative spondylolisthesis). The results showed 9 (75%) of the 12 patients obtained at least a 20% improvement in their preoperative Oswestry score, whereas 6 (55%) of 11 patients with radiographic follow-up achieved a solid fusion by the criteria used in this study. Bridging bone on the anteroposterior film was observed in 10 (91%) of the 11 patients. No systemic toxicity, ectopic bone formation, recurrent stenosis, or other adverse events related to the OP-1 putty implant were observed. A successful fusion was observed in slightly over half the patients in this study, using stringent criteria without adjunctive spinal instrumentation. This study did not demonstrate the superiority of OP-1 combined with autograft over an autograft alone historical control, in which the fusion rate was approximately 55%.

DISCUSSION

Autogenous bone grafting, usually derived from the iliac crest, is frequently used in the treatment of fracture nonunions. The donor-site morbidity and potentially limited supply of suitable autogenous bone are commonly recognized drawbacks. The proven value of reaming by-products, an internal autografting, is quite often inadequate to overcome adverse local circumstances.

Regardless of the ongoing developments of new approaches or the improvement of the current ones for the treatment of fracture nonunions, their management continues to be difficult, even for the more experienced orthopedic surgeons. In addition, there other orthopedic situations dealt in the acute setting or in a more chronic base, where the use of the AICBG alone seems inadequate to overcome the difficulties posed by the local environment. Union rates of different types of nonunions, different degrees of the magnitude of the initial injury, the extent of time between initial injury and final intervention, individual characteristics, multiple previous interventions, and diversities on the application of each biologic enhancement make comparisons and conclusions difficult. On the other hand, recent studies advocated the

benefit and safety of rhBMP-7 or rhBMP-2 in several anatomic sites in nonunions.[13,62,63] Most of the work with BMPs is done on the aseptic long bone nonunion model. It is of interest, however, that recently Chen and colleagues[65] have shown that osteogenic protein-1 (BMP-7) can stimulate new bone formation in the presence of bacterial infection in an intramuscular osteoinduction model in the rat. They speculated that BMPs could eventually be considered as a treatment option to stimulate fracture healing even in the presence of infection and a fixation device and, therefore, earlier removal of the implant and a more timely and effective treatment of the infection could be feasible.

Dimitriou and colleagues[64] have shown 92.3% healing success in 24 of 26 persistent long bone nonunions with the use of graft expansion in these difficult scenarios. Accordingly, Ronga and colleagues[63] in their observational study gave an overall 88.8% healing rate, which showed to be influenced by the number of complications or the number of previous operations (subgroups), once again giving useful information for suggestion of graft expansion in those recalcitrant nonunions. On the contrary, the work of Vaccaro and colleagues[28] in spinal fusion applying the concept of graft expansion without instrumentation shows low healing rates and thus creates considerable skepticism. Nonetheless, the local spinal environment and the lack of instrumentation may explain the differences noted.

The addition of growth factors in AICBG as a graft expansion technique can be considered in situations where the local environment is not favorable for healing. In those situations, this approach of providing a power biologic stimulus in terms of osteogenicity, osteoconductivity, and osteoinductivity appears to be desirable especially in cases

---

Table 3
Properties and consideration of issues for use: autologous cancellous bone graft (ABG) versus bone morphogenetic proteins (BMPs)

Autologous Cancellous Bone Graft	Bone Morphogenetic Proteins
• Biologic method	• Lesser grafting strength compared with ABG
• Osteoconductivity (scaffold)	• Nonbiologic method
• Osteoinductivity	• Osteoinduction
• Viable mesenchymal cells	• No osteoconductivity
• Requires 2nd operation (harvest site)	• No cells
• Limited availability	• Easy of use
• Donor site morbidity	• Ample quantity
	• No donor site morbidity
	• No side effects
	• More expensive

after an already failed autografting procedure for the treatment of fracture nonunions.[63,64] **Table 3** shows the properties of AICBG and BMPs. This approach could not only lower the average number of operations performed but also hospital stay and cost.[2,66] Another scenario for graft expansion with growth factors would be the fracture site with bone loss either circumferentially or as a length defect in the acute setting of trauma or during the aftermath treatment of a nonunion. When a long bone nonunion has been treated with intramedullary nailing in association with a significant bone defect at the nonunion site, the graft expansion principle should be considered. Seemingly, bone defects secondary to extensive debridement, fracture malalignment, or at a later stage (eradication of deep infection, excision of the nonunion site) where an open procedure is about to be performed, represents another potential indication for the concept of graft expansion. Another situation where expansion in the form of percutaneous BMP administration can be considered is a closed exchange nailing procedure for an oligotrophic nonunion where the reaming by-products do not seem adequate as internal grafting to promote healing. In case of serious bone loss, the use of bone graft is an obligatory surgical step.[62–64] However, the number of previous surgical interventions, the extent of the damage to the soft tissue, and the type of previous complications could assist the surgeon toward the choice of the use of autograft in association with BMPs or other biologic active substances and/or implantation of osteoprogenitor cells.

Another area of interest for consideration for graft expansion is the docking site during bone transfer (distraction osteogenesis procedures). Giotakis and colleagues,[66] with regard to the issue of the use of bone graft at the docking site, comment that "if surgeons are asked if bone grafts are used at the docking site,

answers will vary from 'never' to 'always.' This is truer in cases with severe soft tissue damage and atrophic docking ends. However, it is the author's experience that a 'wait and see' approach to docking sites invariably produces extended periods of fixator use, sometimes exceeding the period needed for a regenerate column to consolidate. Nevertheless, bone grafts are not always necessary if docking site clearance and preparation produces two coapted surfaces with contact over a large surface area. Only if contact is poor, bone grafts are mandatory." The possible use of BMPs remains to be seen along with the recreation of the "fresh fracture" at the docking ends.

In **Box 1**, we summarize the possible suggestions for graft expansion with growth factors in various adverse situations.

Regarding the economical burden, Dahabreh and coworkers[2] in a cost analysis of treatment of persistent fracture nonunions, compared the cost implications of treatment of persistent fracture nonunions before and after application of recombinant human BMP-7. Of 25 fracture nonunions, 9 were treated using BMP-7 alone and 16 using BMP-7 and bone grafting. As a final phase of their treatment, the patients were grafted with BMP-7 in all cases, and additional autograft was used in 64%. They concluded that the mean number of procedures per fracture performed before application of BMP-7 was 4.16, versus 1.2 thereafter. The overall cost of treatment of persistent fracture nonunions with BMP-7 was 47.0% less than that of the numerous previous unsuccessful treatments ($P = .001$). They concluded that the early BMP-7 administration in complex or persistent fracture nonunions could reduce significantly the overall cost of treatment.

The same investigation group more recently did a comparative analysis of the cost of treatment of tibial nonunions with either BMP-7 or AICBG. The

---

Box 1
Suggestions for graft expansion with growth factors in various adverse situations

1. Bone loss at the time of injury.
2. Persistent nonunions, when AICBG has failed.
3. Significant bone defect at the nonunion site (greater than 2 cm).
4. More than two previous surgical interventions, extensive damage to the soft tissues, and increased severity of previous complications
5. Presence of bone defect greater than 2 cm after extensive debridement, either initially (open injuries, highly comminuted fractures) or at a later stage (eradication of deep infection, excision of the nonunion site).
6. Exchange nailing to enhance the by-products (injection) especially if the nailing technique was open.
7. Fusion of joints where a defect is substantial and the quantity of AICBG is not sufficient.

authors reported that the average cost of treatment with BMP-7 was 6.78% higher (P = .1) than with AICBG, and most of this (41.1%) was related to the actual price of the BMP-7. In addition to the satisfactory efficacy and safety of BMP-7 in comparison with the gold standard of AICBG, as documented in multiple studies, its cost effectiveness was advocated favorably in this study.

In conclusion, the combined used of AICBG with growth factors (BMPs) can be considered as a powerful biologic stimulus for the treatment of several clinical case scenarios. Certain criteria should be considered for the use of this strategy and for justification of the potential financial implications.

REFERENCES

1. Praemer A, Furner S, Rice DP. Musculoskeletal injuries. In: Barnes, Noble, editors. Musculoskeletal conditions in the United States. Park Ridge (IL): American Academy of Orthopaedic Surgeons; 1992. p. 85–124.
2. Dahabreh Z, Dimitriou R, Giannoudis PV. Health economics: a cost analysis of treatment of persistent fracture non-unions using bone morphogenetic protein-7. Injury 2007;38(3):371–7.
3. Brinker MR. Nonunions: evaluation and treatment. In: Browner BD, Jupiter JB, Levine AM, et al, editors. 3rd edition. Skeletal Trauma Basic science management and reconstruction, vol. 1. Philadelphia: Saunders; 2003. p. 507–604.
4. Blick SS, Brumback RJ, Lakatos R, et al. Early prophylactic bone grafting of high-energy tibial fractures. Clin Orthop Relat Res 1989;(240):21–41.
5. Heiple KG, Goldberg VM, Powell AE, et al. Biology of cancellous bone grafts. Orthop Clin North Am 1987; 18(2):179–85.
6. Johnson KD. Management of malunion and nonunion of the tibia. Orthop Clin North Am 1987; 18(1):157–71.
7. Jones CB, Mayo KA. Nonunion treatment: iliac crest bone graft techniques. J Orthop Trauma 2005;19(10 Suppl):S11–3.
8. Younger EM, Chapman MW. Morbidity at bone graft donor sites. J Orthop Trauma 1989;3:192–5.
9. Cook SD, Wolfe MW, Salkeld SL, et al. Effect of recombinant human osteogenic protein-1 on healing of segmental defects in non-human primates. J Bone Joint Surg Am 1995;77(5):734–50.
10. Paterson DC, Lewis GN, Cass CA. Treatment of delayed union and nonunion with an implanted direct current stimulator. Clin Orthop Relat Res 1980;148: 117–28.
11. Schaden W, Fischer A, Sailler A. Extracorporeal shock wave therapy of nonunion or delayed osseous union. Clin Orthop Relat Res 2001;387:90–4.
12. Friedlaender GE, Perry CR, Cole JD, et al. Osteogenic protein- 1 (bone morphogenetic protein-7) in the treatment of tibial nonunions: a prospective, randomized clinical trial comparing rhOP-1 with fresh bone autograft. J Bone Joint Surg Am 2001; 83:151–8.
13. Giannoudis PV, Tzioupis C. Clinical applications of BMP-7: the UK perspective. Injury 2005;36(Suppl 3):S47–50.
14. Johnson EE, Urist MR, Finerman GA. Resistant nonunions and partial or complete segmental defects of long bones. Treatment with implants of a composite of human bone morphogenetic protein (BMP) and autolyzed, antigen-extracted, allogeneic (AAA) bone. Clin Orthop Relat Res 1992;277: 229–37.
15. Cook SD, Barrack RL, Patron LP, et al. Osteogenic protein-1 in knee arthritis and arthroplasty. Clin Orthop Relat Res 2004;428:140–5.
16. Zhang R, An Y, Toth CA, et al. Osteogenic protein-1 enhances osteointegration of titanium implants coated with periapatite in rabbit femoral defect. J Biomedical Materials Res Part B Appl Biomaterials 2004;71(2):408–13.
17. Mont MA, Jones LC, Elias JJ, et al. Strut-autografting with and without osteogenic protein-1: a preliminary study of a canine femoral head defect model. J Bone Joint Surg Am 2001;83(7):1013–22.
18. Lieberman JR, Conduah A, Urist MR. Treatment of osteonecrosis of the femoral head with core decompression and human bone morphogenetic protein. Clin Orthop Relat Res 2004;429:139–45.
19. Boden SD, Martin GI Jr, Morone MA, et al. Posterolateral lumbar intertransverse process spine arthrodesis with recombinant human bone morphogenetic protein 2/hydroxyapatitetricalcium phosphate after laminectomy in the nonhuman primate. Spine 1999;24(12):1179–85.
20. Cook SD, Dalton JE, Tan EH, et al. In vivo evaluation of recombinant human osteogenic protein (rhOP-1) implants as a bone graft substitute for spinal fusions. Spine 1994;19(15):1655–63.
21. Govender S, Csimma C, Genant HK, et al. BMP-2 Evaluation in Surgery for Tibial Trauma (BESTT) Study Group. Recombinant human bone morphogenetic protein-2 for treatment of open tibial fractures: a prospective, controlled, randomized study of four hundred and fifty patients. J Bone Joint Surg Am 2002;84(12):2123–34.
22. Phieffer LS, Goutet JA. Delayed unions of the tibia. Instr Course Lect 2006;55:389–401.
23. Wiss DA, Stetson WB. Tibial nonunion: treatment alternatives. J Am Acad Orthop Surg 1996;4(5): 249–57.

24. Devnani AS. Simple approach to the management of aseptic non-union of the shaft of long bones. Singapore Med J 2001;42(1):20–5.

25. Souter WA. Autogenous cancellous strip grafts in the treatment of delayed union of long bone fractures. J Bone Joint Surg Br 1969;51(1):63–75.

26. Rodriguez-Merchan EC, Gomez-Castresana E. Internal fixation of nonunions. Clin Orthop Relat Res 2004;419:13–20.

27. Stevenson S. Enhancement of fracture healing with autogenous and allogeneic bone grafts. Clin Orthop Relat Res 1998;355(Suppl):S239–46.

28. Vaccaro AR, Patel T, Fischgrund J, et al. A pilot safety and efficacy study of OP-1 putty (rhBMP-7) as an adjunct to iliac crest autograft in postero-lateral lumbar fusions. Eur Spine J 2003;12(5):495–500.

29. Schmidt AS, Christopher G, Finkemeier CG, et al. Treatment of closed tibial fractures. J Bone Joint Surg Am 2003;85(2):352–68.

30. Wiss DA, Johnson DL, Miao M. Compression plating for non-union after failed external fixation of open tibial fractures. J Bone Joint Surg Am 1992;74(9):1279–85.

31. Weber BG, Brunner C. The treatment of nonunions without electrical stimulation. Clin Orthop Relat Res 1981;161:24–32.

32. La Velle DG. Delayed union and nonunion of fractures. In: Terry Canale S, editor. 9th edition. Campbell's operative orthopaedics. 2. St Louis (MO): Mosby; 1998. p. 579–629.

33. Gershuni DH, Pinsker R. Bone grafting for nonunion of fractures of the tibia: a critical review. J Trauma 1982;22(1):43–9.

34. Boskey AL, DiCarto E, Paschatis E, et al. Comparison of mineral quality and quantity in iliac crest biopsies from high- and tow-turnover osteoporosis: an FTIR microspectroscopic investigation. Osteoporos Int 2005;16(12):2031–8.

35. Heckman JD, Ehter W, Brooks BP, et al. Bone morphogenetic protein but not transforming growth factor-beta enhances bone formation in canine diaphyseal nonunions implanted with a biodegradable composite polymer. J Bone Joint Surg Am 1999;81(12):1717–29.

36. Trueta J. Blood supply and the rate of heating of tibial fractures. Clin Orthop Relat Res 1974;105:11–26.

37. Reed AA, Joyner CJ, Brownlow HC, et al. Human atrophic fracture non-unions are not avascular. J Orthop Res 2002;20(3):593–9.

38. Reed AA, Joyner CJ, Isefuku S, et al. Vascularity in a new model of atrophic nonunion. J Bone Joint Surg Br 2003;85(4):604–10.

39. Bruder SR, Fink DJ, Captan AI. Mesenchymal stem cells in bone development, bone repair, and skeletal regeneration therapy. J Cell Biochem 1994;56(3):283–94.

40. Marsh JL, Buckwalter JA, McCollister-Evarts C. Delayed union, non-union, malunion and avascular necrosis. In: Epps Chang L, editor. Complications in orthopaedic surgery. 3rd edition. Philadelphia: JB Lippincott; 1994. p. 183–211.

41. Mohan S, Baylink D. Chapter 80. Principles of bone biology 1996l;11:11–23.

42. Ring D, Barrick WT, Jupiter JB. Recalcitrant nonunion. Clin Orthop Relat Res 1997;340:181–9.

43. Christensen NO. Kuntscher intramedullary reaming and nail fixation for non-union of fracture of the femur and the tibia. J Bone Joint Surg Br 1973;55(2):312–8.

44. Danckwardt-Lilliestrom G. Reaming of the medullary cavity and its effect on diaphyseal bone. A fluoro-chromic, microangiographic and histologic study on the rabbit tibia and dog femur. Acta Orthop Scand Suppl 1969;12:81–153.

45. Olerud S, Kartstrom G. Secondary intramedullary nailing of tibial fractures. J Bone Joint Surg Am 1972;54(7):1419–28.

46. Reichert IL, McCarthy ID, Hughes SP. The acute vascular response to intramedullary reaming. Microsphere estimation of blood flow in the intact ovine tibia. J Bone Joint Surg Br 1995;77(3):490–3.

47. Utvag SE, Grundnes O, Reikeras O. Graded exchange reaming and nailing of non-unions. Strength and mineralisation in rat femoral bone. Arch Orthop Trauma Surg 1998;118(1–2):1–6.

48. Clancey GJ, Winquist RA, Hansen ST Jr. Nonunion of the tibia treated with Kuntscher intramedullary nailing. Clin Orthop Relat Res 1982;167:191–6.

49. Kempf I, Grosse A, Rigaut P. The treatment of noninfected pseudarthrosis of the femur and tibia with locked intramedullary nailing. Clin Orthop Relat Res 1986;212:142–54.

50. Johnson EE, Marder RA. Open intramedullary nailing and bone-grafting for non-union of tibial diaphyseal fracture. J Bone Joint Surg Am 1987;69(3):375–80.

51. Sledge SL, Johnson KD, Henley MB, et al. Intramedullary nailing with reaming to treat non-union of the tibia. J Bone Joint Surg Am 1989;71(7):1004–19.

52. Wiss DA, Stetson WB. Nonunion of the tibia treated with a reamed intramedullary nail. J Orthop Trauma 1994;8(3):189–94.

53. Megas P, Panagiotopoulos E, Skrivitiotakis S, et al. Intramedullary nailing in the treatment of aseptic tibial nonunion. Injury 2001;32(3):233–9.

54. Reckling FW, Waters CH. Treatment of non-unions of fractures of the tibial diaphysis by posterolateral

cortical cancellous bone-grafting. J Bone Joint Surg Am 1980;62(6):936–41.

55. Wu CC, Shih CH, Chen WJ, et al. High success rate with exchange nailing to treat a tibial shaft aseptic nonunion. J Orthop Trauma 1999;13(1): 33–8.

56. Wu CC. Reaming bone grafting to treat tibial shaft aseptic nonunion after plating. J Orthop Surg (Hong Kong) 2003;11(1):16–21.

57. Johnson EE, Urist MR, Finerman GA. Bone morphogenetic protein augmentation grafting of resistant femoral nonunions. A preliminary report. Clin Orthop Relat Res 1988;230:257–65.

58. Ozkaynak E, Rueger DC, Drier EA, et al. OP-1 cDNA encodes an osteogenic protein in the TGF-beta family. EMBO J 1990;9(7):2085–93.

59. Arrington ED, Smith WJ, Chambers HG, et al. Complications of iliac crest bone graft harvesting. Clin Orthop Relat Res 1996;329:300–9.

60. Fernyhough JC, Schimandle JJ, Weigel MC, et al. Chronic donor site pain complicating bone graft harvesting from the posterior iliac crest for spinal fusion. Spine 1992;17(12):1474–80.

61. Cook SD. Preclinical and clinical evaluation of osteogenic protein-1 (BMP-7) in bony sites. Orthopedics 1999;22(7):669–71.

62. Kanakaris NK, Calori GM, Giannoudis PV, et al. Application of BMP-7 to tibial non-unions: a 3-year multicenter experience. Injury 2008;39(S2):S83–90.

63. Ronga M, Baldo F, Zappala G, et al. Recombinant human bone morphogenetic protein-7 for treatment of long bone non-union: an observational, retrospective, non-randomized study of 105 patients. Injury 2006;37(Suppl 3):S51–6.

64. Dimitriou R, Dahabreh Z, Katsoulis E, et al. Application of recombinant BMP-7 on persistent upper and lower limb nonunions. Injury 2005;36(Suppl 4): S51–9.

65. Chen X, Kidder LS, Schmidt AH, et al. Osteogenic protein-1 induces bone formation in the presence of bacterial infection in a rat intramuscular osteoinduction model. J Orthop Trauma 2004;18(7):436–42.

66. Giotakis N, Narayan B, Nayagam S. Distraction osteogenesis and nonunion of the docking site: Is there an ideal treatment option? Injury 2007;38: S100–7.

Quantitative Analysis of Growth Factors from a Second Filter Using the Reamer-Irrigator-Aspirator System: Description of a Novel Technique

James P. Stannard, MD[a],*, Ashoke K. Sathy, MD[a],
Fariba Moeinpour, MS[a,b], Rena L. Stewart, MD[a],
David A. Volgas, MD[a]

KEYWORDS

- Reamer-Irrigator-Aspirator (RIA) • Bone grafting
- Long bone nonunion • Growth factors • TCP filter

In the United States 7.9 million fractures occur annually. Between 5% and 10% of these fractures result in delayed or impaired healing. More than 1.5 million bone-grafting procedures are performed each year. Iliac crest bone graft has long been considered the gold standard for autogenous bone graft because of its osteoconductive, osteoinductive, and osteogenic properties[1]; however, it is associated with significant donor site morbidity and increased operative time.[2] The Reamer-Irrigator-Aspirator (RIA; Synthes, USA, Paoli, PA) was initially developed to potentially reduce the embolic load associated with reaming the femur for intramedullary nailing in trauma.[3] Subsequently it has been noted that the reamings are biologically active and may provide a source of autogenous bone similar to iliac crest in efficacy, but with fewer donor site complications.[4–10] The RIA system typically uses a single filter to capture the bony reaming debris from the RIA cutting head. Recently it has been noted that the irrigating fluid effluent may also contain significant amounts of growth factors and mesenchymal stem cells.[6,7]

The purpose of this paper is twofold. First, we report on our novel technique of using a second filter containing beta-tricalcium phosphate (TCP) as a graft extender while using the RIA system. Second, we sought to identify whether growth factors known to be present in the bony reaming debris and fluid effluent[6,7,9] are also present in the collections from the TCP filter.

MATERIALS AND METHODS

This study was approved by our Institutional Review Board (IRB). Informed consent was obtained from 16 patients who were prospectively enrolled between February 2007 and May 2007. Inclusion criteria included age older than 19 years and nonunion of a long bone requiring bone grafting; exclusion criterion was active infection at the time of the bone-grafting procedure. Patients

Research funding support for this project was provided by Synthes, Inc, Paoli, PA.
[a] Department of Orthopedics, The University of Alabama at Birmingham, 510 South 20th Street, FOT 950, Birmingham, AL 35294-3409, USA
[b] The University of Alabama at Birmingham, Center for Surgical Research, 1670-University Boulevard, VH G094, Birmingham, AL 35294-0019, USA
* Corresponding author.
E-mail address: james.stannard@ortho.uab.edu (J.P. Stannard).

Orthop Clin N Am 41 (2010) 95–98
doi:10.1016/j.ocl.2009.07.002
0030-5898/09/$ – see front matter © 2010 Published by Elsevier Inc.

could be enrolled if they had a history of prior infection, but no signs of active infection. There were eight males and eight females enrolled with an average age of 40 years (range 22 to 60 years). Seven (44%) of the 16 patients were smokers, 1 (6%) had diabetes, and 9 (56%) had an open fracture with their initial injury. All patients underwent bone harvest and grafting using the RIA system as well as iliac crest aspiration. Samples from the TCP filter were analyzed and compared with the patient's iliac crest bone marrow aspirate.

OPERATIVE RIA TECHNIQUE

Patients were placed supine on a radiolucent table. Bone was harvested using the RIA system through a trochanteric entry portal over a guide wire designed for this system. Access to the trochanteric portal was through a 25- to 30-mm incision that ended approximately 2 cm proximal to the tip of the greater trochanter. The technique is identical to trochanteric intramedullary nailing until the reamer is placed. A threaded wire was placed at the tip of the greater trochanter and drilled into the proximal femur. A cannulated opening reamer was then used to open the proximal femur. A ball-tipped guide wire was then inserted and passed into the distal femur. It is critical to make sure that the guide wire is centered distally. Two 750-µm sterile filters were attached to the suction tubing in series (**Fig. 1**). The reamer head diameter was determined using intraoperative fluoroscopy. The reamer was used in a single-pass fashion using a slow, deliberate advance/withdrawal maneuver. The first filter collected the bony reamings and the second filter contained either large (2.8–5.6 mm) or medium

(1.4–2.8 mm)-sized TCP granules that were washed with aspiration fluid. For all subjects, three stratified (top, middle, and bottom) samples (**Fig. 2**) were taken from the TCP-containing second filter for quantitative analysis of various growth factors. The factors analyzed were vascular endothelial growth factor (VEGF), bone morphogenetic protein-2 (BMP-2), transforming growth factor-beta (TGF-beta), and total protein (TP). Each patient also had iliac crest bone marrow aspirate sent for quantification of these same growth factors. The entry portal was then plugged with a piece of tricalcium phosphate.

PROTEIN AND GROWTH FACTOR ANALYSIS

Samples for total protein analysis were homogenized and centrifuged. Total protein concentration in the supernatant was quantified using the BIO-RAD protein assay kit according to manufacturer protocol. VEGF, BMP-2, and TGF-beta concentration measurements were done using enzyme-linked immunosorbent assay (ELISA) methods from R&D Systems according to manufacturer protocol. Briefly, standards and samples were added to pre-coated plates and incubated. These were then washed with buffer and appropriate conjugates were added and incubated. After another washing these were incubated with the appropriate substrate. Stop solution was then added and the plate was read at the appropriate wavelength.

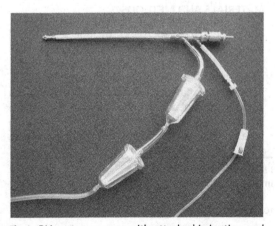

Fig. 1. RIA system reamer with attached irrigation and suction tubing. Filters are in series on suction tubing. Filter 1 captures bony reamings and filter 2 contains TCP granules.

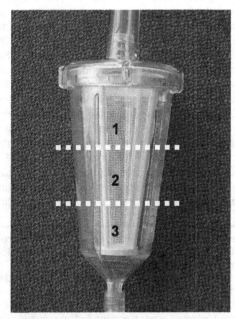

Fig. 2. Filter used in system. Samples were retrieved from the top (1), middle (2), and bottom (3).

STATISTICAL ANALYSIS

Stata 10 (StataCorp, College Station, TX) was used to analyze the data. Visual analysis of the data demonstrated that the data followed a relatively normal distribution, therefore a *t* test was used to compare the mean of the iliac crest bone aspirate with the mean of each sample location for each growth factor.

RESULTS

The concentration of VEGF, BMP-2, TGF-beta, and total protein in the TCP-containing second filter was determined by the ELISA method and compared with the concentration in iliac crest bone marrow aspirate. These data are presented in **Tables 1–4**. The mean concentration of VEGF in TCP (9.26 pg/mg) was significantly lower than that found in iliac crest aspirate (14.38 pg/mg), *P* = .048. BMP-2 was also found at a significantly lower concentration in TCP (10.41 pg/mg) compared with iliac crest (17.01 pg/mg), *P* = .012. TGF-beta was noted at more than double the concentration in TCP (58.58 pg/mg) compared with iliac crest (27.87 pg/mg), *P* = .000. Total protein concentration in TCP (27.68 mg/g) was nearly triple the concentration found in iliac crest aspirate (9.74 mg/g), *P* = .000. Among the three fractions within each TCP filter there did not seem to be any consistent relationship between concentration and location. Granule size did not affect BMP-2, TGF-beta, or VEGF levels collected in the TCP (*P* = .753, *P* = .466, *P* = .509 respectively). A mean of 40 mL of bone graft was obtained with a range of 18 to 55 mL.

DISCUSSION

The RIA is a new system that was initially developed to minimize the potentially harmful pulmonary effects of reaming during intramedullary nailing of femur fractures.[3] Subsequently it has been found to be an alternative method of autogenous bone graft harvest for reconstructive procedures[4,5,8,10] with fewer donor-site complications.[2,4,5,9] The bony reamings harvested using RIA contain osteogenic cells,[6,8] osteoinductive proteins,[7,8] and osteoconductive bony spicules and/or matrix.[8] Newer work suggests that in addition to the actual bony reamings, the irrigating fluid effluent may also contain growth factors and cells that could enhance the overall osteogenic potency of RIA graft. Schmidmaier and colleagues[7] recently demonstrated that both RIA bony reaming debris and the irrigation fluid contain rich amounts of growth factors important in bone formation. They quantified concentrations of platelet-derived growth factor (PDGF), BMP-2, fibroblast growth factors (FGF), VEGF, insulin-like growth factor (IGF-I), and TGF-beta and found a content comparable with that of iliac crest bone graft. Porter and colleagues[6] recently analyzed the cellular component as well as the protein component of RIA filtrate among five patients undergoing hip hemiarthroplasty. They found that the filtrate contains viable mesenchymal stem cells in addition to growth factors such as FGF-2, IGF-I, and TGF-beta1. They suggest that the true osteogenic potential of RIA filtrate may be associated with these musculoskeletal progenitor cells.

To our knowledge we are the first to describe using a second filter filled with TCP to enhance the collection process. This study is part of a larger

Table 2
Bone morphogenetic protein-2, pg/mg

	Mean	SD	P Value
Iliac crest	17.01	7.34	Reference
TCP (top)	11.73	8.83	.103
TCP (middle)	9.31	4.35	.002
TCP (bottom)	10.19	7.26	.014
TCP (mean)	10.41	5.49	.012

Abbreviation: TCP, beta-tricalcium phosphate.

Table 1
Vascular endothelial growth factor, pg/mg

	Mean	SD	P Value
Iliac crest	14.38	11.95	Reference
TCP (top)	8.12	6.00	.031
TCP (middle)	8.46	11.56	.088
TCP (bottom)	11.19	10.07	.168
TCP (mean)	9.26	7.86	.048

Abbreviation: TCP, beta-tricalcium phosphate.

Table 3
Transforming growth factor-beta, pg/mg

	Mean	SD	P Value
Iliac crest	27.87	5.93	Reference
TCP (top)	57.61	20.78	.000
TCP (middle)	67.47	32.43	.000
TCP (bottom)	50.63	19.19	.001
TCP (mean)	58.58	16.35	~.000

Abbreviation: TCP, beta-tricalcium phosphate.

Table 4
Total protein, mg/g

	Mean	SD	P Value
Iliac crest	9.735	1.97	Reference
TCP (top)	32.98	19.82	.003
TCP (middle)	25.31	10.78	.000
TCP (bottom)	24.74	7.37	.000
TCP (mean)	27.679	8.41	~.000

Abbreviation: TCP, beta-tricalcium phosphate.

ongoing investigation into the use of RIA for autologous bone graft harvest. Our initial thought process was to have the TCP serve as an osteoconductive graft extender and to increase the overall volume of the graft harvest. We harvested a mean of 40 mL of graft and then added the TCP to that as a graft extender. This is in keeping with previous reports on graft volume.[4,5,8] We intentionally harvested no more than was necessary, and in all cases we had a sufficient quantity of bone graft. In light of the aforementioned recent work on growth factors in the bony reaming and fluid effluent,[6,7] we also investigated whether these same growth factors are present in the TCP filter. We showed that they are indeed present in substantial amounts. TGF-beta and total protein levels in TCP were higher than in iliac crest aspirate. Although VEGF and BMP-2 levels were lower in TCP compared with iliac crest, significant concentrations were nonetheless present. As part of a larger ongoing study we compared the concentrations of these growth factors in TCP with that in RIA bony reamings and found no statistically significant difference.[9] We did not expect the TCP filter to have equal concentrations of growth factors with the actual bone graft harvested. Neither the size of the TCP granules nor the location within the filter appears to impact growth factor concentrations.

In conclusion, our data indicate that a second filter filled with TCP is not simply a passive osteoconductive graft extender. Our findings imply that significant amounts of additional growth factors can be harvested using a second filter filled with TCP. We believe this is an easy and reproducible modification of the standard RIA technique that could enhance the osteogenic properties of RIA bone graft. Future work could focus on quantifying the amount of viable mesenchymal stem cells in

the second filter filled with TCP. Other areas of research could investigate the impact of using different osteoconductive materials in the second filter. A second filter attached in series with the standard RIA filtration system yields TCP with substantial concentrations of bioactive proteins that are equal to those seen in the bone graft that is harvested in the first filter.

REFERENCES

1. Goldberg VM, Akhavan S. Bone grafts and bone graft substitutes. In: Friedlaender GE, Mankin HJ, Goldberg VM, editors. AAOS monograph series 32. 1st edition. Rosemont (IL): American Academy of Orthopaedic Surgeons; 2006. p. 1–8.
2. Ebraheim NA, Elgafy H, Xu R. Bone-graft harvesting from iliac and fibular donor sites: techniques and complications. J Am Acad Orthop Surg 2001;9: 210–8.
3. Muller CA, Green J, Sudkamp NP. Physical and technical aspects of intramedullary reaming. Injury 2006;37:S39–49.
4. Belthur MV, Conway JD, Jindal G, et al. Bone graft harvest using new intramedullary system. Clin Orthop Relat Res 2008;466(12):2973–80.
5. Newman JT, Stahel PF, Smith WR, et al. A new minimally invasive technique for large volume bone graft harvest for treatment of fracture nonunions. Orthopedics 2008;31(3):257–61.
6. Porter RM, Liu F, Pilapil C, et al. Osteogenic potential of Reaming Irrigator Aspirator (RIA) aspirate collected from patients undergoing hip arthroplasty. J Orthop Res 2009;27(1):42–9.
7. Schmidmaier G, Herrmann S, Green J, et al. Quantitative assessment of growth factors in reaming aspirate, iliac crest, and platelet preparation. Bone 2006; 39:1156–63.
8. Stafford PR, Norris B. Reamer-irrigator-aspirator as a bone graft harvester. Tech Foot Ankle Surg 2007; 6(2):100–7.
9. Stannard JP, Volgas DA, Stewart RL, et al. Autograft bone graft harvest using an intramedullary reamer. Poster presented at: Orthopaedic Trauma Association 23rd Annual Meeting. Boston (MA), October 17–20, 2007.
10. Weatherby B, Norris BL, Nowotarski P, et al. Reamer irrigator aspirator (RIA) bone graft harvesting in nonunion and segmental defect repair. Poster presented at: American Academy of Orthopaedic Surgeons Annual Meeting. San Diego (CA), February 14–18, 2007.

RIA: One Community's Experience

Christopher G. Finkemeier, MD, MBA[a],*, Rafael Neiman, MD[b],
Domingo Hallare, MD[c]

KEYWORDS

- Reamer • Irrigation • Aspiration • Fat embolism
- Nonunion • Autologous • Bone graft • Morbidity

The patients discussed in this article were all treated at a level 2 community trauma center located in a suburb of a moderately sized city and serves a community of 1 million persons. With only a few exceptions, the authors are the only users of the Reamer Irrigator Aspirator (RIA) at our hospital. All the authors are fellowship-trained orthopedic trauma surgeons and have practices that are approximately 85% acute trauma and 15% reconstructive and elective general orthopedics. The authors work directly with the general trauma surgeons on the trauma service and have a separate call schedule from the general orthopedic surgeons. The trauma service has an average of 1200 trauma admissions per year. The authors began using RIA in 2003 and, as in many of the centers using RIA shortly after its release, the authors primarily used RIA for the acute treatment of femur and tibia fractures in polytrauma patients with chest injury or with two or more long bone fractures. The general trauma surgeons were highly influential in convincing the hospital of the importance of RIA for our severely injured patients with long bone fractures.

As experience and early reports were disseminated about the benefits of RIA as a bone-harvesting instrument, we began to use RIA increasingly more as a bone graft harvesting tool. The authors have been reluctant to abandon autologous bone graft in favor of the ever-increasing array of bone graft substitutes because of our belief that autologous bone with all of its bone-promoting components is ideal for bone healing. This core belief in addition to the low donor site morbidity of RIA seen in our patients has made RIA-harvested bone graft our graft of choice for most reconstructive surgeries not requiring structural properties.

INDICATIONS

Our group has three main indications for RIA: harvesting of nonstructural bone graft, treating acute or chronic intramedullary infection, and intramedullary nailing of multiple long bone fractures or in patients with a chest contusion and one or more long bone fractures.

In our practice, the most common indication for RIA is for bone graft harvesting. We believe that autologous bone graft is the best bone graft for most bone-healing applications. Because the graft material obtained with RIA is a granular material with varying degrees of gelatinous consistency, it is not useful as a structural graft. Tri-cortical iliac crest or allograft blocks are better suited for this purpose. However, if bone graft material is needed for healing of bone defects, nonunions, and so forth, autologous bone graft harvested with RIA is our first choice. We believe that cortical-cancellous bone harvested from the medullary canal of femurs provides a bone graft with osteogenic, osteoconductive, and osteoinductive properties.[1–3] Given the minimal morbidity with harvesting this rich bone graft using RIA, we prefer it to

[a] Orthopedic Trauma Surgeons of Northern California, Sutter Roseville Medical Center, 5897 Granite Hills Drive, Roseville, CA 95746, USA
[b] Orthopedic Trauma Surgeons of Northern California, Suite 1005, Roseville, CA 95661, USA
[c] Department of Orthopedics, Orthopedic Trauma, Kaiser Permanente South Sacramento, 6600 Bruceville Road, Sacramento, CA 95823, USA
* Corresponding author.
E-mail address: finkemeier@surewest.net (C.G. Finkemeier).

Orthop Clin N Am 41 (2010) 99–103
doi:10.1016/j.ocl.2009.07.007

demineralized bone matrix, bone morphogenic proteins, solid allograft preparations, or combinations of these materials. We cannot rationalize using bone graft substitutes in an attempt to mimic autologous bone graft when we can harvest the real thing with little risk and morbidity to the patient. In addition, the volume of graft obtained with RIA can be abundant but can also be voluntarily adjusted to need based on reamer size. On the other hand, the volume of graft harvested with RIA may be limited because of patient age (osteopenia) and systemic diseases that affect bone quality.

Although not one of the early applications of RIA, we have used RIA as a tool to debride and irrigate the medullary canals of long bone infections. We have used RIA in both the femur and tibia and believe that it can debride the entire medullary canal and irrigate and remove the infectious material in an efficient single technique. The suction/aspiration feature of RIA minimizes pressurization of the canal, which theoretically decreases or eliminates dissemination of the infected material deeper into the cortical bone or into the circulation.

As alluded to earlier, we still use RIA in selected acute long bone fractures. Because of anecdotal reports of increased nonunion rates in acute fractures, we do not use RIA for isolated femur fractures. Although this nonunion concern is unproven and unsubstantiated, we do not feel there is any advantage to RIA for acute femoral nailing in isolated femur fractures; however, if a patient with a femur fracture has a significant pulmonary contusion, we would choose to use RIA in an effort to decrease or eliminate marrow embolism. The other acute fracture indication is in patients with bilateral femur fractures with or without associated tibia fractures. However, we have not used RIA in patients with lung injury or multiple long bone fractures in the past 2 years mainly because of our practice of damage control orthopedic procedures (provisional external fixation with delayed intramedullary nailing) in these at-risk and borderline patients. Because the negative effects of marrow embolism associated with reaming of tibia fractures are not as clearly defined as they are in reaming of the femur fractures, we do not feel that RIA is indicated for acute tibia fractures associated with pulmonary injury. The technique of RIA in tibias is much more difficult because the smallest reamer size is 12 mm and because of the eccentric starting point and relatively acute turn that the reamer needs to make in the proximal tibia. The rigid 5 to 6 cm at the tip of the RIA and semi-rigid tube reduces the flexibility of the RIA and increases the chance of a complication when used in the tibia. However,

with a retro-patellar entry point technique, these complications may possibly be eliminated. We have not used retro-patellar technique to date, but we would consider it if we decided we needed to use RIA in the tibia.

TECHNIQUE OF HARVESTING INTRAMEDULLARY BONE WITH THE REAMER IRRIGATOR ASPIRATOR

RIA-harvested bone graft is obtained through a system that incorporates a nitinol drive shaft, a single-use sharp reaming head, and a disposable plastic tube. The components are assembled in a manner that allows the delivery of a cooling irrigant, usually 0.9% normal saline, through the center portion of the nitinol shaft and out through the center port of the reamer head through gravity feed. While spinning in a high-speed, low-torque manner, the reamings become mixed with the irrigant solution and are aspirated through several ports in the sides of the reamer head, out through the plastic tube that surrounds the drive shaft, and into an inline collection filter.

When choosing a starting point for obtaining RIA graft, we consider several options. We often choose an ipsilateral site when harvesting for a lower extremity graft to minimize immobility. When femoral RIA harvesting is used for upper extremity grafts, the desire of the patient is taken into consideration (ie, right versus left), when possible. In aseptic nonunions of the femur, after hardware has been removed, that same ipsilateral femur may be harvested to obtain graft, with the understanding that the yield may be lower. The tibia is not usually used for obtaining graft for concern of thinning the posterior cortex as the bone is harvested, although it has been used on multiple occasions for debridement of endosteal infection within the tibia, where the leg is supported by splinting or other means after debridement.

Hence, we obtain most RIA graft harvestings from the femur, through one of four different starting points. Proximal starting points consist of the piriformis fossa and the greater trochanter, with a larger number of trochanteric start points for ease of manipulating the stiff plastic/nitinol assembly, ease of obtaining the starting point correctly, and with the perception that the trochanteric cortical bone is thinner and cancellous bone more abundant than the piriformis region, yielding more graft from the proximal femur. These two sites mirror those starting points used for antegrade femoral nailing. The distal femoral sites are either an extra-articular medial starting point, chosen to avoid violating the knee joint anterior and proximal to the insertion of the medial collateral ligament,[4] or an intra-articular site anterior to the anterior cruciate ligament (ACL), in a manner identical to our retrograde femoral nailing entry point.

We position the patient supine on a radiolucent table, and use the fluoroscope to confirm the proper starting point and assist with determining reamer head size. With proximal femoral stating points, we place a small bump under the ipsilateral hip before sterile skin prep, and adduct the leg to ease insertion. To determine reamer head size, we place a radiolucent measurement guide (Synthes, Paoli, PA) against the side of the diaphysis, near its isthmus, at the same level as the bone. If placed on top of the thigh or leg, the body habitus of the patient may make the distance from the bone to the skin large enough to introduce error owing to differences in magnification. Depending on how much bone is anticipated to be required, we choose a reamer 1 to 2 mm larger than the endosteal canal width. The thickness of the cortex must be taken into account, so as not to introduce risk of fracture by overthinning of the cortex, especially with older patients.

We then introduce a 3.2-mm guide pin into the site and advance it enough to allow passage of a cannulated, fluted 6.0- to 10.0-mm step drill (Synthes). Once the canal is entered, we introduce a 2.5-mm ball-tipped reaming rod and confirm a center placement at the distal end by fluoroscopy, or in cases of multiple passes, we direct it toward the desired area of metaphyseal bone in one or the other femoral condyle. We pass the reamer slowly down the intramedullary canal in an "advance-withdraw" technique, where the reamer is advanced several centimeters, then withdrawn slightly, then advanced again, until reaching the opposite end of the canal. We take care to monitor the outflow of irrigant through the tube to ensure suction is not lost by clogging within the tube, which could cause malfunction of the RIA system or potentially harm the graft. This occurs commonly in younger patients with dense bone. We collect the reamings, but the effluent irrigant solution is not currently retained. Reamings are kept in a sealed container until use.

APPLICATION OF THE GRAFT/WHEN WE USE ADJUNCTS

After preparation of the site for bone grafting, we place the RIA graft similar to other autologous bone grafts. RIA graft has a consistency similar to moist sawdust. We recommend irrigating the wound before application of the graft to minimize loss, as the graft is not solid and could wash away if exposed directly to would irrigation. We use the RIA graft to fill voids in nonunion sites as well as in acute lengthening. The soft tissue adjacent to the graft should be healthy, and direct contact between the fracture/osteotomy site, RIA graft, and muscle is preferable. When the handling characteristics of the RIA graft are not ideal for that particular application, we manipulate it in one of two ways. If enough volume is present, we can compress it by placing it into a 30- or 60-mL syringe and compact it with the plunger, rendering the plug more dense. In the case of older patients, where yield is unexpectedly low or with high fat content, we may supplement the RIA graft with demineralized bone matrix (DBX, Synthes) to improve volume or improve handling characteristics, so that the graft is more likely to remain where placed.

PITFALLS

Several circumstances can result in complications postoperatively. Pain is the leading complaint after RIA, and this resolves quickly in most patients. Some of our patients had virtually no pain at the RIA harvest site; however, on occasion, pain did linger. Some patients formed a hematoma at the harvest site, although none required surgical drainage. This has led us to attempt sealing of the entry portal using a thickened version of an absorbable gelatin hemostatic agent (Surgifoam, Johnson and Johnson, Cincinnati, OH), which is mixed as a thick paste and deposited into the entry portal. Consistently delivering the absorbable hemostat to the entry portal has been difficult, but can best be controlled when we fill a 15-cm section of leftover RIA tubing with the agent, place it into the entry portal, push the agent through the tube with a solid rod, and remove the plastic tube.

When making multiple passes with RIA, we are careful not to breach the far-sided cortex. This could result in pain or iatrogenic fracture. In one case where the patient had prolonged knee pain after antegrade RIA harvesting, MRI revealed no cortical violation but intense extra osseous edema adjacent to the lateral femoral epicondyle. This has discouraged us from redirecting the guide wire in multiple sites in the distal femur. As mentioned, our experience with RIA in the tibia has been limited to reaming for acute fractures and infection; both circumstances require stabilization of the tibia regardless of the reaming procedure, while neither circumstance provided the confidence for obtaining bone graft. The femur is longer, with more opportunity for harvesting cancellous bone along with the cortical bone, and as such is our preferred long bone for harvesting.

The multiple literature reports of hip and knee pain after femoral fracture with intramedullary nailing demonstrate inconclusive evidence regarding the superiority of a specific entry portal.[5–8] Knee pain can exist after antegrade nailing, whereas hip pain can occur after retrograde nailing. Piriformis and trochanteric starting sites have been shown to have similar incidences of hip pain Our group of patients did demonstrate hip pain that rapidly resolved, leading us to conclude that perhaps other factors associated with the traumatic injury to the femur or the instrumentation of the femur are more responsible for chronic hip pain than the reaming of the proximal femur.

There are several unpublished reports of fracture of the femur occurring after RIA harvesting in the femur and tibia, although none in our series. Care must be taken to avoid eccentric reaming of the proximal cortex of the femur or tibia, or in the case of the distal femoral extra-articular start, the distal lateral femur. Reamer head size must be chosen carefully, and with a small diameter canal, RIA may not be appropriate, as it is currently available only from 12 mm and larger. Osteoporosis is a relative contraindication for RIA harvesting if no internal instrumentation or protection from weight bearing follows the harvest, as the risk of fracture would be unacceptably high.

Results

Over an 18-month period, from June 2005 to December 2006, we performed 23 procedures requiring the use of the RIA. There were 13 males and 10 females. Nineteen procedures were for treating nonunions, two for malunions, two for polytraumatized patients with pulmonary injuries, and one for osteomyelitis. Of the nonunions, seven were in the tibia, four were in the femur, five were in the humerus, one was in the radius, one was in the ulna, and one was in the pelvis. There were 13 males and 10 females. The average age of the patients was 50 years (range 21 to 77 years). Of the two patients who had malunions, both were in the femur. Both required acute femoral lengthenings and derotation osteotomies. Of the two polytraumatized patients who had pulmonary injuries, one patient had a femur shaft fracture, and the other had both femur and tibia shaft fractures. One patient had tibial osteomyelitis.

In most cases, RIA was used in the femur shaft entering the proximal femur in antegrade fashion through a trochanteric entry portal. In the other cases, RIA was used in the tibial shaft, from the medial femoral condyle, or in the femur in a retrograde fashion. In the cases where RIA was used to harvest bone, variable amounts of harvested bone were obtained, ranging from 20 mL to more than 100 mL.

To investigate the morbidity of RIA, we retrospectively reviewed our cases in which RIA was used in the femur via an antegrade approach with a trochanteric starting point. Fifteen patients were able to be identified who met these criteria. The morbidity was assessed using the Oxford hip score as an outcome measure. The Oxford hip score is an outcome instrument that assesses hip pain by using a 12-item questionnaire. The minimum total score of 12 points indicates normal function and the maximum score of 60 indicates severe disability.[9] This was modified to grade responses as *excellent* if the final score fell between 12 and 27, *good* if the score was between 28 and 43, and *poor* if the final score was between 44 and 60. The average Oxford hip score for these patients was 15.8 (range 12 to 27), indicating an excellent result.

After the initial study period, we have performed 14 procedures using RIA: 2 cases were infections and 12 cases were nonunions.

Complications

During our initial study period, we had three complications. The first was a failure to achieve union in a distal tibial nonunion. The patient required a second procedure, which included harvesting bone graft from the contralateral femur using RIA. The patient healed after the second procedure. The second complication was in a patient with a femur malunion. He had complaints of medial-sided knee pain in the distribution of the saphenous nerve. This had subsided at last follow-up. Our third complication was an infection of the distal tibia and ankle. This patient had an open fracture and tibial infection after her index procedure. RIA was used in her tibia to harvest bone graft for an ankle arthrodesis. Four months after her ankle arthrodesis, she presented with erythema and purulent drainage necessitating repeat debridements and removal of hardware. Her multitude of problems included avascular necrosis of the talus, recurrent ankle infection, and nonunion of the ankle and subtalar joints. She chose amputation as definitive treatment.

SUMMARY

RIA is a successful implement for the harvesting of large volumes of nonstructural autologous bone graft. It provides an osteogenic, osteoinductive, and osteoconductive environment for bone healing. It is easy to learn, as many surgeons are already familiar with the technique for intramedullary nailing. Once beyond the "learning curve," harvesting with RIA takes less time than traditional autologous iliac crest harvesting. RIA is highly effective in promoting the healing of nonunions and segmental defects, including acute lengthenings. It can also be used for treatment of endosteal long bone infections of the tibia and femur. The complication rate for RIA harvesting is lower than that expected for harvesting of autologous iliac crest graft, although it is not without risk, especially if reamer size is too aggressive, reaming technique is indiscriminant, or bone quality is poor. Its contribution to chronic hip pain appears to be minimal. In our community trauma practice, RIA has replaced iliac crest bone grafting as the autologous graft of choice for nonstructural defects and nonunions.

REFERENCES

1. Frolke J, Nulend J, Semeins C, et al. Viable osteoblastic potential of cortical reamings from intramedullary nailing. J Orthop Res 2004;22:1271–5.

2. Wenisch S, Trinkaus K, Hild A, et al. Human reaming debris: a source of multipotent stem cells. Bone 2005; 36:74–83.

3. Hoegel H, Mueller C, Peter R, et al. Bone debris: dead matter or vital osteoblasts. J Trauma 2004;56: 363–7.

4. Swiontkowski M, Hansen S, Kellam J. Ipsilateral fractures of the femoral neck and shaft. A treatment protocol. J Bone Joint Surg Am 1984;66(2): 260–8.

5. Bain GI, Zacest AC, Paterson DC, et al. Abduction strength following intramedullary nailing of the femur. J Orthop Trauma. 1997;11:93–7.

6. Ricci W, Schwappach J, Tucker M, et al. Trochanteric versus piriformis entry portal for the treatment of femoral shaft fractures. J Orthop Trauma 1996; 20(10):663–7.

7. Ricci WM, Bellabarba C, Evanoff B, et al. Retrograde versus antegrade nailing of femoral shaft fractures. J Orthop Trauma 2001;15:161–9.

8. Ostrum RF, Agarwal A, Lakatos R, et al. Prospective comparison of retrograde and antegrade femoral intramedullary nailing. J Orthop Trauma 2000;14: 496–501.

9. Field R, Cronin M, Singh P. The Oxford hip scores for primary and revision hip replacement. J Bone Joint Surg Br 2005;87:618–22.

Managing Bone Deficiency and Nonunions of the Proximal Femur

John J. Perry, MD[a],*, Brent Winter, MD[b], Jeffrey W. Mast, MD[c]

KEYWORDS
- Nonunion • Subtrochanteric • Femur • Nail
- Plate • Revision

Fractures of the peritrochanteric and subtrochanteric region of the femur can represent a significant problem in the primary setting. In the revision setting, dealing with bone loss and correcting deformity increases the difficulty. These fractures have large mechanical forces exerted over very short bone segments. Koch described the forces acting on the proximal femur and observed that a 100-lb force could create 1250 lb/in^2 of compression on the medial side of the femur and 1000 lb/in^2 of tension on the lateral side of the femur.[1] These forces have a significant impact on the treatment of proximal femur fractures and, to overcome them, durable implants that attain reliable fixation are needed. Current primary treatment of these factures has shifted from plate osteosynthesis to that of intramedullary splinting. Several intramedullary devices have been developed with enlarged proximal bodies and large screws that insert into the femoral head to overcome the deforming forces of these fractures, sometimes referred to as cephalomedullary nails. Some studies suggest these larger implants can provide increased initial stability. A study by Roberts and colleagues found that the fracture site motion was decreased in unstable subtrochanteric fractures with implants designed as cephalomedullary nails have large proximal bodies.[2] Although the development of new implants has lead to improved stability over older extramedullary implants, it is not without cost. The amount of bone removed from the proximal femur is significantly increased when compared with plate fixation and can lead to problems of implant dependency and bone voids and problems during revision of these implants in ununited or malunited fractures. The tremendous forces acting on the proximal femur are compounded when there is little bone for implants to obtain purchase. In the setting of nonunions and malunions of the proximal femur, the bone defects typically need to be addressed.

Despite these drawbacks, the prevailing treatment has shifted to intramedullary nails with cephalic locking options. Biomechanical studies comparing intramedullary fixation and plate fixation are conflicting. A study by Tencer and coworkers found an advantage in intramedullary nailing with respect to combined bending and compression, although plates and intramedullary constructs were able to support at least 100% of a human's body weight.[3] A more recent

a Mammoth Orthopedics and Sports Medicine, PO Box 3834, Mammoth Lakes, CA 93546, USA
b 3336 South Pioneer Parkway Suite 102, West Valley City, UT 84120, USA
c Mammoth Orthopedics and Sports Medicine, Sierra Park Orthopedics, PO Box 660, Mammoth Lakes, CA 93546, USA
* Corresponding author.
E-mail address: jperry1014@aol.com (J.J. Perry).

Orthop Clin N Am 41 (2010) 105–118
doi:10.1016/j.ocl.2009.08.001
0030-5898/09/$ – see front matter © 2010 Elsevier Inc. All rights reserved.

biomechanical study showed increase displacement in an unstable subtrochanteric fracture model with use of the gamma nail (Stryker, Kalamazoo, Michigan) compared with a 95° angle blade plate (Synthes, Paoli, Pennsylvania).[4]

Initial treatment of these fractures is difficult, regardless of the implant chosen for fixation. Forces on the proximal femur tend to externally rotate, flex, and abduct the proximal fragment, and correction of these forces is critical for the initial treatment of these fractures to be successful. Anatomic reduction is the best way to insure appropriate healing of these fractures at the initial time of surgery and affords patients the best opportunity to gain full recovery. Anatomic reduction is imperative for normal hip kinematics and to promote rapid union. A durable implant, like a cephalomedullary implant, placed poorly that can induce malreduction cannot always be relied on to attain final union. If union is attained, then a residual deformity may leave a patient with a deformed extremity, altered gait, or limp

The rate of symptomatic malunion is rarely reported in the literature.[5] Wiss and Brien defined malunion as shortening greater than 1 cm, 10° of angulation in any plane, or rotational malalignment greater than 15°. They reported six malunions out of 98 subtrochanteric femur fractures treated with intramedullary nailing.[6] Malunion can be severely disabling with shortening of the affected extremity or persistent limp that does not improve without surgical intervention.

Despite the reported increased biomechanical favorability of intramedullary implants used to treat proximal femur fractures, the affect of these large implants has not been studied. The enlarged proximal body implants remove a significant amount of cancellous bone in the head, neck, and peritrochanteric region of the femur that is difficult to replace in revision surgery. Volumetric analysis of three popular cephalomedullary implants ranges from 21 to 27 cm³ (**Table 1**). Subsequent removal of these implants, therefore, exemplifies the problem surgeons must anticipate when dealing with these large defects. Not only is the bone loss large but also it is directly in the region of the compression and tension trabeculae of the proximal femur, which are of utmost importance in hip structural integrity.

The rate of nonunion of the subtrochanteric femur fracture healing is reported as between 1% to 20% in the orthopedic literature. Few studies have been done looking at revision surgery of subtrochanteric nonunions. Options include revision to a larger intramedullary implant, fixation with a plate, or hip arthroplasty with typically a calcar replacing implants in older patients with severely diminished bone stock. Haidukewych and Berry reported on 23 nonunions that underwent revision using a variety of implants, including cephalomedullary nails and blade plates.[7] Twenty of the 21 nonunions healed and two were lost to follow-up. Eighteen of the 23 required additional bone grafting. The investigators concluded that different implants can be used successfully depending on fracture location and bone quality; however, statistically significant differences could not be found with the limited numbers of patients.

de Vries and colleagues[8] evaluated results of subtrochanteric nonunions treated with blade plating techniques. Thirty-two of 33 nonunions healed with this technique. They thought that blade plates were more suited for nonunions with deformity, as anatomic correction and compression with the plate is reliable whereas use of intramedullary implants is challenging and limited. They also emphasized key steps in treating these nonunions: correction of malalignment, bone grafting when necessary, and internal fixation with compression. Barquet and colleagues reported on a series of 26 patients with subtrochanteric nonunion treated with revision surgery with

Table 1
Volumetric analysis of cephalomedullary nails

	Nail Description	Nail Volume (cm³)	Blade/screw Description	Blade/screw Volume (cm³)	Sleeve (cm³)	Total Volume (cm³)
TFN	11 mm × 130°, 170-mm long	15.96	110 mm long	6.65	n/a	22.61
Gamma	11 mm × 130°, 180-mm long	15.84	75 mm long	3.86	n/a	19.70
IMHS	12 mm × 130°, 210-mm long	19.91	105 mm long	4.83	2.30	27.04

Abbreviations: IMHS, intramedullary hip screw; n/a, not applicable; TFN, trochanteric femoral nail.
Data courtesy of Synthes, Paoli, Pennsylvania.

a long cephalomedullary nail. Their results were good, with 88% going on to union after one procedure and 25 of 26 uniting after additional procedures, including nail dynamization and bone grafting.[9] They chose to use a gamma nail due to the biomechanical advantage, allowing immediate postoperative weight bearing, and because of the large proximal body that filled the proximal bone defects. They reported six patients with continued varus deformity greater than 5° postoperatively, three of whom had a pre-existing varus deformity that was not corrected. Correction of deformity and compression across the nonunion site are difficult to attain with a cephalomedullary nail during revision surgery. In the authors' experience, the majority of proximal femoral nonunions have residual deformity that typically needs to be addressed at the time of revision to assure union and restoration of normal gait.

The revision of intramedullary fixation of the proximal femur is a technically demanding surgery, which requires significant preoperative planning. Surgical tactics must allow for contingency plans for problems typically encountered during the procedure. In addition to bridging large cavitary bone defects with biomechanically stable fixation, surgeons must promote reconstitution of bone loss to allow later implant removal. Recent advances in reaming techniques and harvesting of osteoinductive, autogenous cancellous grafts combined with established uses of structural, osteoconductive allografts allow consistent management of these two problems.

In the authors' experience, proximal femoral fracture nonunions and malunions with bone loss are best treated with four typical steps: first, removal of previous hardware; second, bone grafting of defects; third, controlled osteotomy to correct deformity and restore normal anatomy; and fourth, and finally, attaining a stable, load-sharing construct by tensioning the implant and using Association for the Study of Internal Fixation (ASIF) techniques, thereby compressing the osteotomy and allowing early weight bearing and rapid bone consolidation.

Preoperative planning is required to deal with proximal femoral fractures with bone loss. Included in this planning are identification of the previous implant and having any special equipment required for removal, the need for and degree of osteotomy, having structural allograft and the ability to obtain autogenous bone graft for osteoinduction, and, finally, the ideal implant for controlled reduction and definitive stabilization. A preoperative workup for infection is also important. This usually consists of erythrocyte sedimentation rate, C-reactive protein, and a white blood cell count. A preoperative plan with templating of the corrective osteotomy level, including the degree and the steps of the procedure, should be visible to the entire operating room team. This helps prevent confusion and allows everyone to know the current step and next step in the operative plan by reviewing the surgical tactic.

In most situations, an extensile approach to the hip is used through a lateral approach. The tensor fascia lata aponeurosis is split longitudinally and the vastus lateralis is freed laterally and transversely at the inferior aspect of the vastus ridge and elevated anteriorly with a posterior based L-shaped incision. Only the lateral side of the femur is dissected free; preserving the vascular supply to medially based fragments is paramount. In cases of atrophic nonunions, the nonunion site is débrided until punctuate bleeding from both ends is encountered. In this case, more extensive exposure of medial based structures may be needed. In hypertrophic nonunions where stability at the fracture site is the main cause of nonunion, a thorough débridement is not necessary.

Removal of failed hardware is usually the first step in dealing with these revision surgeries. Correction of deformities is impossible without removing the failed previous implants. Prevention of further bone loss is important in these difficult fractures. Having the proper equipment available can help to remove implants in an efficient and atraumatic manner. Most implants have removal devices that minimize further iatrogenic injury and should be made available. A broken screw removal set aids in removal of broken hardware. In the most difficult situations, a metal cutting burr can be beneficial in freeing and extracting incarcerated hardware. The time required for this initial part of the procedure should not be minimized.

The authors' technique of managing the resultant bone defects is multifaceted. Bone grafting depends on the size and extent of the bone loss. In general, use of structural allograft is imperative for increasing strength of the fixation in the head and blocking loss of cancellous graft from the large peritrochanteric defects. The authors typically use preshaped allograft cortical bone dowels stacked sequentially into the screw/head defect and then dowels that block egress of cancellous graft from the holes left by the nail in the trochanter, lateral femur, and subtrochanteric canal (**Fig. 1**). Alternatively, cortical struts or matchsticks can sometimes be used in the screw/head defect. Cancellous graft is liberally impacted into the open proximal femur and around the interstices of the allograft.

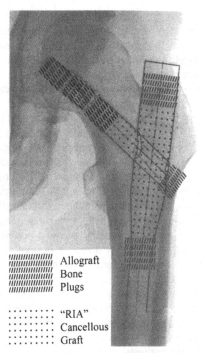

Allograft
Bone
Plugs

"RIA"
Cancellous
Graft

Fig. 1. Preshaped allograft cortical bone dowels are stacked sequentially into the screw head defect to augment blade plate fixation. Dowels are then placed in the trochanter, lateral femur, and subtrochanteric canal to stop egress of cancellous graft from the holes left by the nail.

The large cancellous defects left in the peritrochanteric region require generous amounts of osteoinductive, cancellous autograft. Traditionally, autogenous graft was harvested from the ipsilateral iliac crest through a separate incision and then morselized and impacted into the defects. This requires an additional incision and has been associated with additional complications, including prolonged pain, infection, hematoma, and even lateral femoral cutaneous nerve palsy. Iliac crest bone graft can provide limited volumes from some crests that can be insufficient for the large defects encountered. The authors use the Reamer-Irrigator-Aspirator System (RIA, Synthes) to harvest morselized bone graft from the ipsilateral femoral canal after the previous hardware is removed.[10] Recent studies suggest the advantage of this system in that it is a negative pressure system that minimizes embolic phenomena and irrigates the canal, minimizing thermal injury that may be induced with standard reamers and reaming techniques.[10] The aspirated graft shares many of the growth factors and delivers comparable

amount of osteoconductive and inductive tissue compared with iliac crest grafting techniques with less morbidity.[11] This technique allows obtaining large volumes, in excess of 30 cm³, of rich cancellous graft typically in excess of what is required with little or no added morbidity or surgical time. The reamer head selected is at least 2 mm larger than the implant removed. A guide rod is bent and the advanced down, alternating sides of the distal femur passing the RIA after the guide rod has been repositioned. Fibular strut allografts have been shown to provide a reliable, biologic structural support in the postoperative period and, over time, partially incorporates with the surrounding native bone.[12,13] First, a fibular strut allograft or cortical dowels are used to fill in the hole left in the head from the cephalic screw. Secondly a dowel or plug is used to block the femoral canal at the level of the lesser trochanter; thirdly dowel is placed in the superior greater trochanter defect. Filling the holes allows having an impact the copious amounts of morselized autograft obtained with the RIA. The lateral hole left from the entrance of the cephalic screw can then be blocked with another dowel or with the blade plate itself to keep the autograft from displacing. The authors' technique, as depicted in **Fig. 1**, has afforded a reliable way to improve fixation in the femoral head of the definitive implant while at the same time restoring the large volumes of bone stock destroyed by the previous enlarged proximal body of the cephalomedullary device. Residual graft can also be placed around the nonunion or osteotomy site before final closure.

Although replacing existing bone defects is an important part of a successful plan in treating peri- and subtrochanteric nonunions, it cannot be overemphasized that correction of the typical biomechanical and biologically unfavorable varus and shortened deformity is paramount for success. Having multiple implants available to obtain fixation, while allowing correction of deformity in these fractures, can be useful. The use of revision reconstruction nailing provides satisfactory results,[9] but there are several drawbacks to using them. It is difficult to obtain correction of the deformity of the previous fracture with an intramedullary nail. As discussed previously, correction of the deformity is an essential step in revision surgery of the proximal femur and, in some cases, correcting this deformity and changing the biomechanical forces is enough to provide an ideal biologic environment for healing. The nail is also not as amendable to intraoperative contouring to optimize correction as the blade plate. Intramedullary nailing can also makes future surgery of the proximal femur even more difficult as additional bone is removed to seat the implant or a new hole is created to correct malalignment.

The question of whether or not to débride the nonunion site, complete the osteotomy through the nonunion, or fish scale the area is purely academic. The questions are, at which level is the osteotomy done and which angle is more relevant. Typically, the authors bypass the nonunion site and complete the controlled osteotomy at a lower level for several reasons. First, most nonunions of this area are due to poor stability or poor biomechanics and deformity, leading to hypertrophic or oligotrophic nonunions. Oligotrophic nonunion is rare and may suggest infection, osteonecrosis secondary to thermal necrosis from overzealous reaming, or significant devascularization. Secondly, nonunions lack distinct sharp edges and dense cortical bone that when compressed with the plate store energy well and impart stability. Thirdly, bypassing the nonunion avoids causing further devascularization of the nonunion. Finally, a controlled osteotomy at a lower level allows for longer proximal segment that can be more easily controlled and compressed.

The orientation of the osteotomy must take into consideration restoration of normal anatomy and leg length. Sometimes a double-level osteotomy is anticipated if greater than 2 cm of lengthening is required (**Fig. 2**). Typically, the osteotomy is short and oblique, allowing easy correction of the common malrotation while also allowing the more simple correction of flexion, extension or varus, or valgus deformities. Lengthening of 1 cm can typically be obtained through a single-level osteotomy (discussed later). The sharp short edges are ideal for obtaining excellent stability in multiple planes once the plate is tensioned.

In the authors' experience, implants that can provide rigid fixed-angle fixation in the proximal fragment and compression at the osteotomy or nonunion site are the most suitable implants. Many newer implants exist that can be used for revision surgery in the proximal femur and they each have advantages and disadvantages. The workhorse implant for this reconstruction, in the authors' experience, is the well-established blade plate. The angled blade plate is a commonly used implant in revision surgery of the proximal femur. It has been used for many years with reliable results in primary and revision surgery involving the proximal femur.[14] It allows for reproducible correction of malunions or nonunions when appropriate preoperative planning is performed and executed. Opponents of the blade plate state that it is a technically difficult implant to use as it must be inserted in the correct

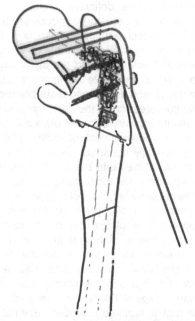

Fig. 2. Depicts two short oblique osteotomies below the captured proximal segment of a nonunion that can then allow translation of the intecallary segment laterally to facilitate gaining leg lengths approaching 2 cm.

orientation in all three planes for it to be used successfully. The authors, like other proponents of its use, find that in the hands of surgeons familiar with its use and with tissue-friendly techniques, it allows tremendous intraoperative flexibility with reliable and proved results. This implant can be bent intraoperatively, afford impaction of auto and allograft bone to impart proximal segment stability, allows correction of the deformity, and final compression of the nonunion or osteotomy site in one construct.

Understanding the proper use of the plate mandates understanding that placement of the initial seating chisel as the pivotal point of the procedure. An appropriately placed seating chisel that results in the correction of the multiplanar deformity, as determined by the preoperative plan and intraoperative fluoroscopy once the osteotomy is completed, is the pivotal point of the procedure. If a surgeon cannot identify the multiaxis deformity and the appropriate placement of the seating chisel that will reverse these deformities in the preoperative plan and then later in surgery, then failure results. With the angled blade plate, the surgeon impacts the auto/allograft into the head and gains an idea of the quality of fixation in the head before definitive fixation with the implant. Once the osteotomy is completed, after appropriate placement of the seating chisel, capture of the proximal fragment is obtained with the definitive blade plate and the distal fragment is then fixed to the plate using an articulating tension device and articulating plate clamps. This provides compression at the osteotomy, creating a load-sharing construct for the plate and bone.

The recent development of locked plating to create fixed-angle constructs is an alternative to using angled blade plate but the authors do not commonly use it for most complex reconstructions. The proximal femoral locking plate and proximal femoral hook plate incorporate this technology. These plates may be inserted more easily than a blade plate and allow for multiple points of fixation in the proximal femoral segment. These implants may be more easily adjusted than the blade plate if placed in an improper orientation. The disadvantage of the proximal femoral locking plate is that it requires a longer proximal bone segment for fixation compared with the blade plate and, therefore, is not appropriate in many situations. Osteotomies can be performed before its insertion in similar fashion to the blade plate technique and the plate is pretensioned using the articulating tension device.

In cases of short proximal fragments with an intact greater trochanter, the proximal femoral hook plate can be used. The hook plate is a large fragment plate with two proximal hooks that capture the superior tip of the greater trochanter and resists varus angulation of the proximal femur. Additionally, two locking screws can then be placed into the femoral head to provide a fixed-angle construct in the proximal fragment. This implant has the same advantages of the proximal femoral locking plate but adds the potential of capturing the greater trochanter. The addition of the hooks supports more effective application of tension to the plate by including the greater trochanter in the construct. It is then fixed to the distal fragment and tensioned, compressing the osteotomy in a load-sharing capacity with an articulated tensioning device. The disadvantage of these newer plates is their inability to have an impact on already deficient bone in the head and neck region, as the blade plate can. Also, these plates do not allow for use of a seating chisel and its advantages (discussed previously) before completing the definitive osteotomy. Compared with the blade plate, little literature has substantiated these newer devices' efficacy in treating malunions and nonunions of the proximal femur.

Having multiple implants available and a preoperative plan for each implant use completed before the procedure allows adjustment intraoperatively when difficulties are encountered. The authors typically complete three preoperative plans with the three fixed-angle plate constructs (as previously discussed in this paper). The underlying biomechanical tenets are the same for all three implants. Use of a fixed-angle device to capture the proximal fragment and tensioning of the plate, thereby compressing the osteotomy or nonunion by using an articulated tensioning device, is essential for providing a stable environment for healing and early rehabilitation. Three cases illustrate the authors' technique in managing these difficult cases.

CASE 1

A 50-year-old healthy woman presented after five failed surgical procedures to obtain union from an initial three-part reverse obliquity subtrochanteric femur fracture. Her initial procedure was blade plate fixation, which subsequently failed. She next underwent conversion to a cephalomedullary nail. Despite dynamization of the nail and bone marrow aspirate injections, she experienced a painful limp with a perceived leg length discrepancy. Subsequent radiographs confirmed persistent nonunion (**Figs. 3** and **4**).

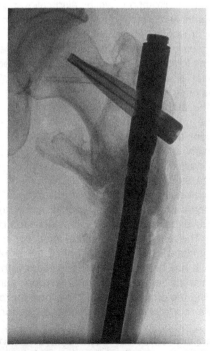

Fig. 3. AP hip radiograph showing nonunion of 50-year-old female as described in Case 1.

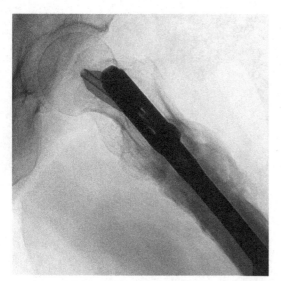

Fig. 4. Lateral hip radiograph showing nonunion of 50-year-old female as described in Case 1.

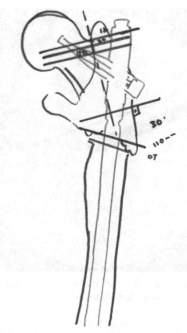

Fig. 6. Depicts a short oblique osteotomy which allows excellent compression and rotational correction and easily affords access to the subtrochanteric canal for grafting.

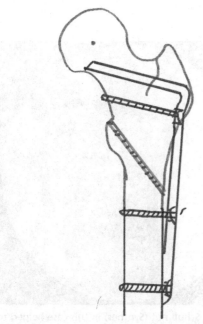

Fig. 5. Depicts an alternative plan for a long oblique osteotomy that may allow good mismatch of the osteotomy surfaces therefore improving stability but would not allow rotational correction.

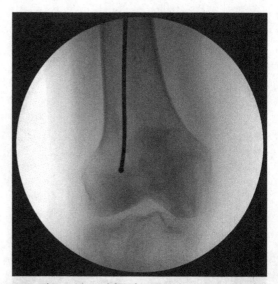

Fig. 7. The guide rod for the RIA is bent and placed in the distal femur to obtain reamings from both condyles.

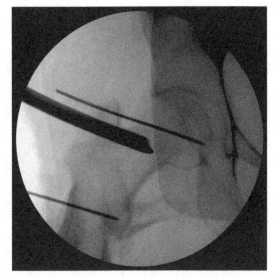

Fig. 8. AP hip floroscan demonstrating guide pin placement and seating chisel advancements.

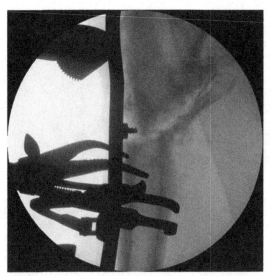

Fig. 10. The plate is reduced to the shaft thereby correcting the deformity and then the osteotomy is compressed with the articulated tensioning device.

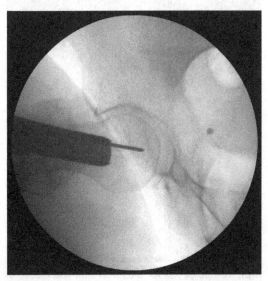

Fig. 9. Lateral hip floroscan demonstrating guide pin placement and seating chisel advancement.

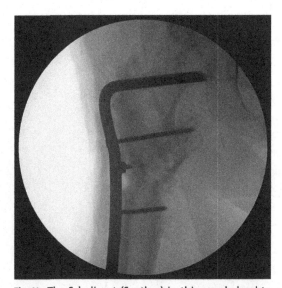

Fig. 11. The Schuli nut (Synthes) in this case helped to fine tune the valgus angulation by acting as a blocking screw. The Schuli nut can also be used to convert a nonlocking screw to a locking screw in the plate if desired due to bone quality.

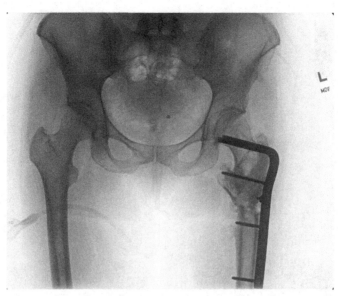

Fig. 12. Case 1. Postoperative radiographs confirm reduction comparable to the preoperative plan.

Preoperative CT scanogram confirmed a 0.5-cm leg length discrepancy and radiographs confirmed the typical varus, shortened extended deformity. Surgical team members designed different preoperative plans with different implants (**Figs. 5** and **6**) and the surgical plan depicted in **Figure 1** was selected. **Fig. 5** demonstrates a longer oblique closing wedge osteotomy through the nonunion site, which would be difficult to compress and provide the stability required for rapid healing and rehabilitation. The long obliquity would also make it more difficult to correct rotational deformities. **Fig. 6** demonstrates a short osteotomy through good bone below the nonunion that can easily be compressed. This allows correction of multiplane deformity and compression of the nonunion at the same time without further devascularization to the nonunion site. Surgical execution begins with exposure and removal of the failed implant. The guide rod for the RIA is bent and placed in the distal femur to obtain reamings from both condyles (**Fig. 7**). Allograft plugs are then placed in the proximal femur as depicted by (see **Fig. 1**) and proximal void left by the large proximal body of the nail is filled. Guide pins are advanced for the osteotomy (see **Fig. 6**) and seating chisel placement and then the chisel is impacted (**Figs. 8** and **9**). The chisel is removed and the osteotomy below the nonunion is preformed. The blade plate is impacted. The plate is reduced to the shaft with an articulating plate clamp and the osteotomy is compressed with the articulating

tension device (**Fig. 10**). The Schuli nut (Synthes) used in this case helped to fine-adjust the valgus angulation as a blocking screw (**Fig. 11**). The Schuli nut can also be used to convert a nonlocking screw to a locking screw in the plate if desired

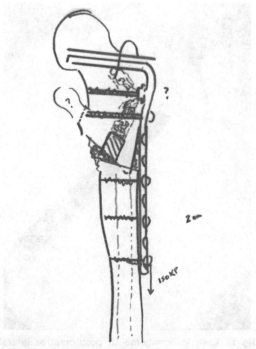

Fig. 13. Postoperative radiographs (see **Fig. 12**) confirm reduction comparable to the preoperative plan.

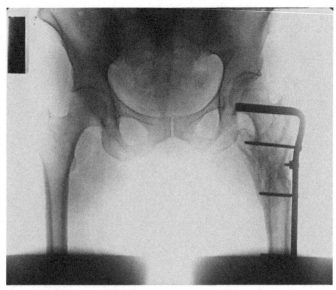

Fig. 14. Case 1. Twenty-month postoperative AP pelvis radiograph confirms union of both nonunion and osteotomy sites.

due to poor bone quality. Postoperative radiographs confirmed reduction comparable to the preoperative plan (**Figs. 12** and **13**). Twenty-month follow-up radiographs confirmed union of the osteotomy and nonunion site (**Figs. 14** and **15**).

CASE 2

A 29-year-old healthy man sustained a four-part intertrochanteric femur fracture. He was subsequently treated with a cephalomedullary nail at a level one trauma center. After 1 year he complained of continued limp, pain, and the hip feeling

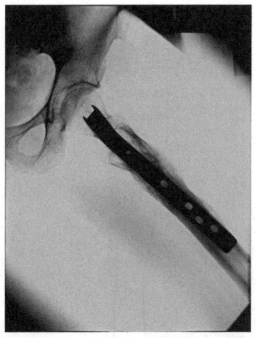

Fig. 15. Case 1. Twenty-month postoperative lateral radiographs confirm union of both nonunion and osteotomy sites.

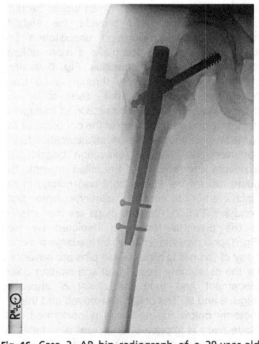

Fig. 16. Case 2. AP hip radiograph of a 29-year-old male with painful nonunion and limp.

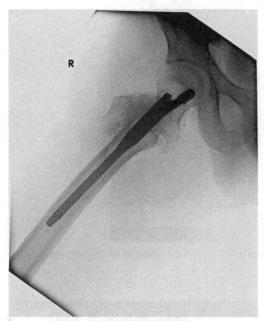

Fig. 17. Case 2. Lateral hip radiograph of a 29-year-old male with painful nonunion and limp. Notice extension deformity.

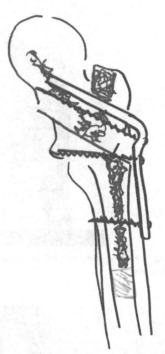

Fig. 19. Case 2. Preoperative plan to correct varus and shortening encountered after initial failed treatment with cephalomedullary nail and bone grafting as described. The long oblique osteotomy also allows a long surface area for mismatch compression.

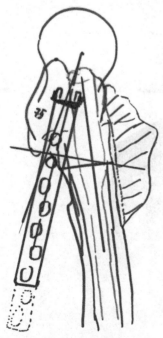

Fig. 18. Demonstrates the preoperative plan that corrects the significant sagittal plan deformity that can be seen when treating nonunions encountered after initial treatment of proximal femur fractures with cephalomedullary nails.

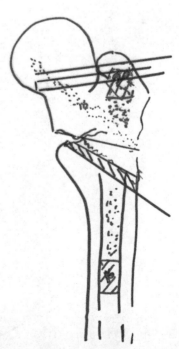

Fig. 20. Allograft dowels and RIA grafting are planned to fill the proximal defects left by the nail.

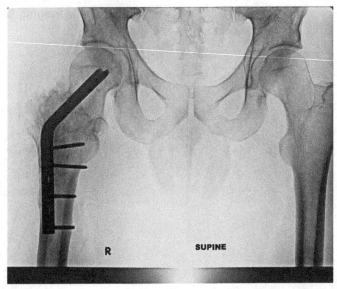

Fig. 21. Case 2. Nineteen-month AP pelvis radiograph confirms union with restoration of length and valgus angulation of the neck.

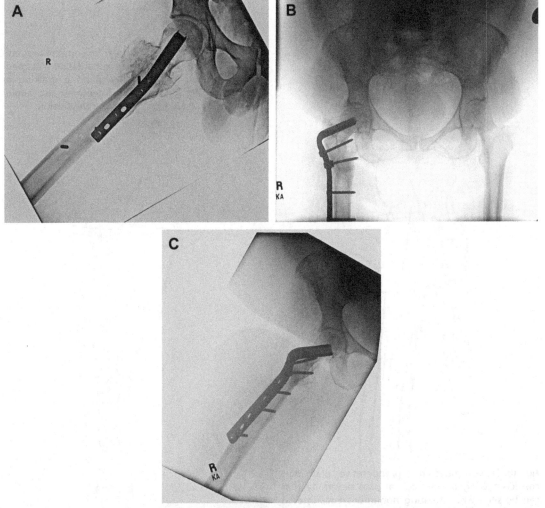

Fig. 22. (*A*) Case 2. Nineteen-month lateral hip radiograph confirms union with correction of extension deformity. (*B*) Case 3. One-year AP pelvis radiograph confirms union with restoration of length and proximal femoral geometry. (*C*) Case 3. One-year lateral hip radiograph confirms union and proximal femoral geometry.

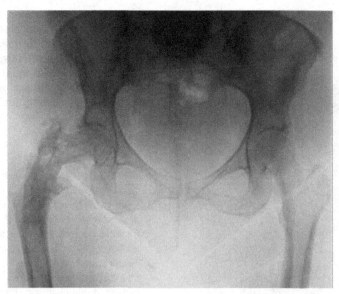

Fig. 23. Case 3. A 57-year-old female with deformity after removal of an infected cephalomedullary nail.

"not in the normal place" (**Figs. 16** and **17**). Preoperative CT scan showed a shortening of seven millimeters and significant flexion deformity. Preoperative planning with an angled blade plate allows adding length through the osteotomy (**Figs. 18** and **19**). Allograft plugs and RIA grafting were planned to fill the proximal defect (**Fig. 20**). Nineteen-month follow-up radiographs confirmed union and the patient has no complaints of pain and feels as though he walks normally again (**Figs. 21** and **22**A).

CASE 3

A 57-year-old disabled obese smoker with diabetes presents with a grossly deformed leg after failure of a cephalomedullary implant and subsequent infection requiring removal of implants leaving her with disabling pain and inability to bear weight (**Fig. 23**). Adduction/abduction radiographs suggest correct ability (**Figs. 24** and **25**). Preoperative studies suggested no residual infection. Preoperative plan was executed (**Fig. 26**). One-year follow-up confirmed union and the patient was ambulatory with a walker and without pain (**Figs. 22**B and **22**C). This case exemplifies that with proper biomechanics are restored during the procedure and using recent grafting techniques, healing can be obtained in even a difficult patient like this.

Revision surgery of the proximal femur with bone loss is difficult under the best circumstances. It requires an understanding of biomechanical forces acting on the femur and using these forces advantageously. Correcting deformity and using load-sharing devices provide for a stable construct for healing. Bypassing the area of nonunion with a controlled osteotomy at a lower level that can then be compressed with a fixed-angle plate allows rapid healing of osteotomy and nonunion. Having all the proper equipment and supplies available is essential to performing this surgery well. Autologous and allogenic bone graft should be available to fill in bone defects and nonunion sites. Multiple implants should be available to adjust to the bone

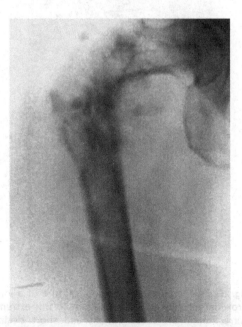

Fig. 24. Functional views include abduction radiographs to suggest correctability.

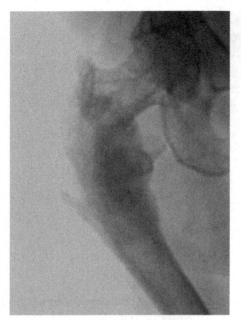

Fig. 25. Functional views include adduction radiographs to suggest correctability.

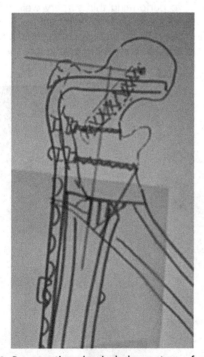

Fig. 26. Preoperative plan includes capture of a long proximal segment to ensure stability in this extreme correction in an obese patient and short closing wedge osteotomy for correction and ease of compression.

defects that are encountered. A preoperative plan is paramount to aid in preparation. Although these nonunions are difficult to treat, the authors have found that with proper planning, surgical execution with proved techniques, and the addition of newer graft harvesting techniques, anatomic restoration and bone healing is nearly assured.

REFERENCES

1. Koch JC. The laws of bone architecture. Am J Anat 1917;21:177–298.
2. Roberts CS, Nawab A, Wang M, et al. Second generation intramedullary nailing of subtrochanteric femur fractures: a biomechanical study of fracture site motion. J Orthop Trauma 2002;16(3):231–8.
3. Tencer AF, Johnson KD, Johnson DC, et al. A biomechanical comparison of various methods of stabilization of subtrochanteric fractures of the femur. J Orthop Res 1984;2:297–305.
4. Bredbenner TL, Snyder SA, Mazloomi MS, et al. Subtrochanteric fixation stability depends on discrete fracture surface points. Clin Orthop Relat Res 2005;432:217–25.
5. Parker MJ, Dutta BK, Sivaji C, et al. Subtrochanteric fractures of the femur. Injury 1997;28:91–5.
6. Wiss DA, Brien WW. Subtrochanteric fractures of the femur: results of treatment by interlocking nailing. Clin Orthop Relat Res 1992;283:231–6.
7. Haidukewych GJ, Berry DJ. Nonunion of fractures of the subtrochanteric region of the femur. Clin Orthop Relat Res 2004;419:185–8.
8. de Vries JS, Kloen P, Borens O, et al. Treatment of subtrochanteric nonunions. Injury 2006;37:203–11.
9. Barquet A, Mayora G, Fregeiro J, et al. The treatment of subtrochanteric nonunions with a long gamma nail. J Orthop Trauma 2004;18:346–53.
10. Nichols TA, Sagi HC, Weber TG. An alternative source of autograft bone for spinal fusion: the femur:technical case report. Neurosurgery 2008; 62(3):E179.
11. Schmidmaier G, Herrmann S, Green J, et al. Quantitative assessment of growth factors in reaming aspirate, iliac crest and platelet preparation. Bone 2006;39(5):E1156–63.
12. Buecker PJ, Gehardt MC. Are fibula strut allogrants a reliable alternative for periarticular reconstruction after curretage for bone tumors? Clin Orthop Relat Res 2007;461:170–4.
13. Enneking WF, Campanacci DA. Retrieved human allografts: a clincopathological study. J Bone Joint Surg Am 2001;83:971–86.
14. Kinast C, Bolhofner BR, Mast JW, et al. Subtrochanteric fractures of the femur: results of treatment with a 95 degree condylar blade-plate. Clin Orthop Relat Res 1989;238:122–30.

Soft Tissue and Biomechanical Challenges Encountered with the Management of Distal Tibia Nonunions

Ivan S. Tarkin, MD*, Peter A. Siska, MD, Boris A. Zelle, MD

KEYWORDS

- Distal tibia • Nonunions • Malunion bone graft
- Bone morphogenetic protein • Soft tissue management

An individualized plan of care is of paramount importance when faced with the challenge of managing nonunion of the distal tibia. Successful reconstruction of distal tibia nonunion is predicated on precisely manipulating the local biomechanical milieu to encourage osseous healing. The unique soft tissue constraints and difficult mechanical environment of the lower leg provoke thoughtful consideration of treatment options for any particular host and nonunited fracture.

Nonunion after fracture of the distal tibia is not an uncommon event. Failure of bone healing is greater than 5% after the index operative procedure.[1] Patients diagnosed with distal tibia nonunion frequently are affected profoundly in terms of their physical, mental, and emotional well-being. These patients have significant challenges returning to both their vocational and social lives. Thus, it is of paramount importance to stop the cycle of disability by instituting a well-organized treatment strategy directed at achieving bony union and promoting physical function.

Coincident with the theme of this issue on bone grafting strategies for fracture care, most nonunions of the distal tibia are atrophic, oligotrophic, or variants with bone loss. These often require biologic supplementation to achieve uneventful union. Bone grafting should be considered an integral part of the overall reconstructive strategy.

TENUOUS SOFT TISSUE ENVIRONMENT

Prerequisites for uneventful healing of distal tibia nonunion include optimizing mechanics at the fracture site while respecting the often tenuous surrounding soft tissue envelope. The soft tissue sleeve adjacent to the nonunited fracture has unique characteristics that must be taken into consideration during the planned reconstructive effort. Proper soft tissue management is often predictive of treatment success or failure.

In the uninjured state, the distal leg has a very limited biologic potential because of the paucity of muscular coverage. At least a third of the distal tibia circumference is subcutaneous in location. In the injured state, the quality of soft tissue coverage overlying the distal tibia is even further compromised. Frequently, these fractures are the result of high energy trauma resulting in irreversible damage to the soft tissue sleeve,[2] which is compounded by previous attempts at surgical fracture care.

COMPROMISED VASCULARITY

In addition to the quality of the soft tissue envelope surrounding the nonunited distal tibia, the status of the local vascularity must be considered in the work-up and eventual plan for reconstruction. Etiology for the development of nonunion may be

Department of Orthopedic Surgery, Division of Traumatology, University of Pittsburgh, 3471 Fifth Avenue, Suite 911, Pittsburgh, PA 15213, USA
* Corresponding author.
E-mail address: tarkinis@upmc.edu (I.S. Tarkin).

Orthop Clin N Am 41 (2010) 119–126
doi:10.1016/j.ocl.2009.07.009
0030-5898/09/$ – see front matter © 2010 Elsevier Inc. All rights reserved.

inherent in the poor local blood supply to the distal tibia from the prior trauma, previous surgery, or host disease (**Fig. 1**). When designing future approaches for nonunion care, the local vasculature needs to be understood and respected to avoid complications such as wound problems, infection, and continued nonunion.[3]

Arterial injury is correlated with the development of tibial nonunion.[4,5] It has been shown that a significant percentage of high-energy distal tibia fractures have occult injury to the arterial tree of the leg. Using computed tomography angiography, an incidence of more than 50% has been reported with the anterior tibial circulation being the most often involved.[6] It is expected that open fractures have an increased risk of occult arterial injury.

Further insult to the local vasculature can occur when open plating is performed at the index operation. Typically, disruption of the intraosseous blood supply occurs with the initial fracture. Thus, the periosteal network is of increased importance for fracture healing. Latex injection studies have demonstrated that open plating techniques can adversely affect the remaining extraosseous blood supply to the metaphysis of the distal tibia.[7]

BIOMECHANICAL CHALLENGES

After taking into account the management of the tenuous soft tissue envelope and the local vascularity, a well-coordinated strategy needs to be used to improve the local mechanical environment of the bony anatomy. In most cases, revision internal fixation and sometimes deformity correction will be necessary to encourage uneventful bony healing of distal tibia nonunion (**Fig. 2**). Although a variety of different fixation and reduction techniques can be used, the preoperative plan must be designed to the unique personality of the nonunion and host.

Aside from the choice of hardware used, there are many factors to consider that are unique to nonunion of the distal tibia. Achieving adequate distal fixation is crucial, but sometimes a significant challenge. In many circumstances, there is a short distal segment. Thus, the corridor for hardware placement is a challenge. Moreover, the bony architecture in the metaphyseal/epiphyseal region is largely cancellous and the distal block is often weakened by disuse osteopenia and previous hardware installation.

In addition to achieving sufficient fixation, correction of deformity is integral to the overall success of reconstruction as defined by bony union and improved functionality. Deformity is commonplace after initial treatment for these fractures with reported rates of 16% after intramedullary nailing and 13% after plate osteosynthesis.[1] Thus, the individualized plan of care must be designed to address restoration of the mechanical/anatomic axis of the tibia when warranted.

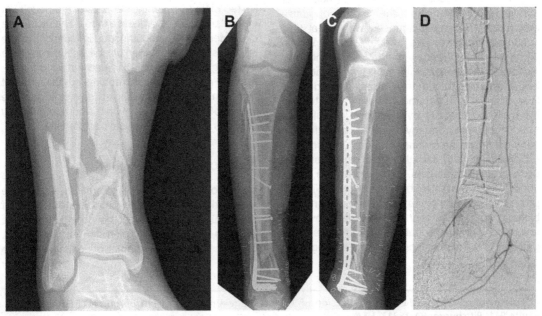

Fig. 1. Delayed union of high-energy open fracture of distal third tibia (*A*) treated with debridement flap, and minimally invasive plate osteosynthesis (*B, C*). Causes for delayed healing were multifactorial including open fracture, vascular insufficiency, poor nutrition (polytrauma patient), tobacco abuse. (*D*) Angiogram demonstrates arterial injury to the anterior and posterior tibial circulation.

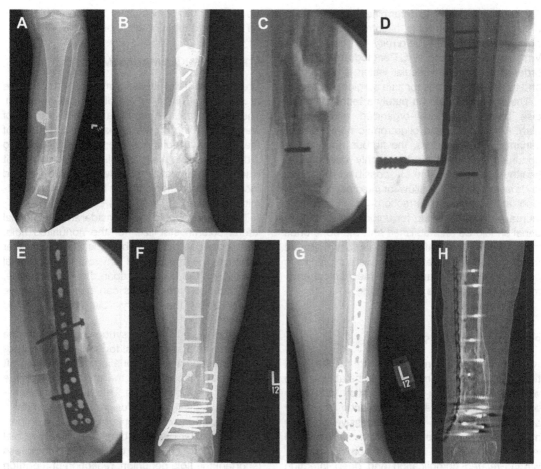

Fig. 2. Preoperative radiograph of oligotrophic distal tibia nonunion with varus deformity (*A, B*). Precise alignment of the anatomic/mechanical axis of the tibia achieved after debridement of the nonunion scar (*C*) and corrective fibular osteotomy (*D*). Peri-articular locking plate used to assist in deformity correction and for rigid fixation of the short osteopenic distal segment. Fibula rigidly fixed and used as biologic lateral column support. Compression of nonunion with interfragmentary compression (*E*). Central bone graft technique used. Patient healed at 4 months (*F–H*).

BIOLOGIC REQUIREMENTS

All distal tibial nonunion variants except hypertrophic or infected cases require biologic supplementation. Therefore, a critical step for achieving osseous healing in atrophic/oligotrophic nonunions or cases with significant bone loss is the delivery of biomaterials to the fracture site. These materials optimally are osteoconductive, osteoinductive, and osteogenic. Osteoconductive biomaterials will serve as a scaffold for new bone growth across the nonunited fracture, whereas osteoinductive and osteogenic agents will stimulate the formation of new bone.

PRINCIPLES OF NONUNION CARE

The unique characteristics of distal tibial nonunion have been discussed. The treatment algorithm

prescribed must be custom tailored to the specific patient and nonunion variant. General principles of nonunion care, however, are applicable to these patients/nonunions.[8]

Although these reconstructive surgeries are not entirely elective cases, a sufficient amount of time should be devoted to counseling the patient and preoperative planning. A contract needs to be made between surgeon and patient outlining the expectations for continued limb salvage. The patient's general wellness both physically and psychologically needs to be maximized. Negative behaviors such as tobacco or alcohol use should be curtailed. Consideration for endocrine work-up should be considered to determine potential systemic etiology contributing to nonunion.[9]

At a minimum, infection should be worked up as a potential cause of nonunion with laboratories,

A CT scan is valuable to determine the pattern and type of nonunion (atrophic, oligotrophic, hypertrophic, nonunion with deformity or bone loss). Vascular studies such as CT angiogram could be ordered if treatable vascular lesion is suspected and to determine areas for safe surgical exposure.

The surgery should be purely a technical exercise based on a well-organized preoperative plan. For atrophic and oligotrophic nonunions or variants with bone loss, the fibrous scar at the nonunion needs to be thoroughly debrided to healthy-appearing bone. If possible, the bone ends are manicured to allow for maximal compression and deformity correction. In an effort to increase surface healing for union, the medullary canal should be reestablished and the bone ends "feathered." Bone graft is packed into and around the nonunion site. Strategic hardware is placed to obtain and maintain an optimal mechanical environment to encourage bone healing.

PLATE OSTEOSYNTHESIS

An integral part of nonunion surgery for the distal tibia is addressing mechanical instability. The workhorse is revision internal fixation with plate osteosynthesis; however, a balance must be achieved. Injudicious use of excessive or bulky hardware in a compromised soft tissue envelope leads to a multitude of severe complications.[10] Wound-related complication and deep infection infamously plague this type of reconstruction. Further, excessive bone stripping during open procedure often can foster continued nonunion.

Fixed angle plates are ideally suited for definitive reconstruction of distal tibia nonunion. Classically, the blade plate has been used with clinical success as defined by union and improved functionality.[11–15] Reduction and compression of the nonunion is facilitated with the use of this implant. Fixation of the short osteopenic distal segment is optimized. However, technical expertise with these devices is warranted for treatment success.

Another option for increasing fixation of the compromised distal segment is with precountoured locking implants. Low profile plates are available for use anterolaterally, medially, and posteriorly. Implant design allows for the placement of multiple fixed angle screws into the distal segment to invite increased control over the nonunited fracture. Further, deformity correction is often facilitated by using the plate as a template for restoring the geometry of the distal tibia. Compression at the site of nonunion can be achieved with eccentric screw placement in the shaft through the dynamic compression slots.

Additionally, an articulating tension device can be applied to most of these plates.

STRATEGIC FIBULA MANAGEMENT

Creative use of the fibula can increase the chances of successful union of the distal tibia nonunion. The fibula can be manipulated in a variety of ways depending on the management strategy of the associated tibial nonunion. When developing a definitive strategy for the distal tibia nonunion it is important to realize that the fibula can be used mechanically, biologically, or to assist with deformity correction.

The fibula should be considered a potential lateral column stabilizer for the nonunited tibia. The fibula can act as a biologic plate to further enhance the mechanical environment for tibial healing. As the fibula will span the nonunion site, syndesmotic type screws can be placed above and/or below the primary tibial fracture line to enhance stability.[16]

The fibula and adjacent syndesmotic membrane can serve as a perfect host for bone graft incorporation creating a single bone leg distally. The graft is typically placed under the muscular envelope overlying the syndesmosis. This vascularized environment is ideally suited for graft incorporation.[17]

Manipulation of the fibula is of utmost importance for either gaining compression of the tibial nonunion or for correcting deformity. To compress (shorten) the tibia nonunion, resection of a portion of the fibula or oblique slide osteotomy is often required. Correction of deformity in the coronal or sagittal plane is exceedingly difficult without simultaneously correcting fibula deformity. As the fibula will often heal, strategic osteotomy needs to be considered.

INTRAMEDULLARY NAILING

Considering the tenuous soft tissue envelope of the distal leg, reamed intramedullary fixation of distal tibia nonunion is an attractive option. This technique is familiar to most orthopedic surgeons and can be performed using minimally invasive methods. The reaming process is integral to the success of this procedure. Reaming serves to debride the fracture nonunion of interposed fibrous tissues. Bone graft is generated and deposited at the site of nonunion. The process of reaming restimulates the inflammatory cascade for bone healing.[18] A fracture hematoma rich in bone morphogenic protein and growth factors is established. Last, reaming enlarges the internal diameter of the distal tibia to accommodate a larger intramedullary implant consequently improving the local mechanics at the nonunion site.

The primary indication for nail fixation is for nonunion in the face of a retained intramedullary rod. The merits of exchange nailing for distal tibia nonunion are evidenced by optimal union rates with an acceptable rate of complication in selected patients.[19] As compared with open plating strategies, the risk of local complication is minimized as direct exposure of the nonunion site in the previously traumatized soft tissue envelope is frequently unnecessary. The risk of wound-related complication including deep infection is decreased. The local vascularity required for bone healing is preserved when the adjacent muscular envelope and periosteum is not disrupted surgically.

Despite the attractiveness of intramedullary nailing, this strategy is not the panacea for the management of all distal tibia nonunions. Nonunion personality must dictate whether this strategy is optimal. The individualized plan of care must consider whether a rod will sufficiently change the local biomechanics toward uneventful healing.

Obtaining and maintaining fixation in a short often osteopenic distal segment is a concern with intramedullary fixation of these nonunion. A nail has the potential to "swim" in the capacious distal segment, which creates instability at the nonunited fracture leading to continued nonunion or possibly malunion. However, nail design has evolved to increase distal fixation. In most modern nails, there are multiple options for locking in different planes. The last locking hole has been moved more distally. Further, the newest designs have incorporated fixed angle technology for the distal locking bolts.

RING FIXATORS

Although not the authors' preferred method of treatment, the Ilizarov fixator is ideally suited for certain distal tibia nonunion variants. A Type C host with a compromised soft tissue envelope would benefit from external fixation as the primary mode for nonunion site stability. Slow correction of substantial deformity is best served with a ring fixator. Massive bone loss requiring bone transport should be managed with a frame.[20] Last, infected cases are best served with Ilizarov technique versus internal fixation.[21]

When choosing Ilizarov techniques, patient selection is key, as responsible frame use and care is mandatory for successful outcomes. Pin tract infection leading to osteomyelitis is the most concerning complication of frame usage.[22]

Patient tolerance and satisfaction with use of these devices is variable.

BIOLOGIC SUPPLEMENTATION STRATEGIES

Most distal tibia nonunions will benefit from biologic supplementation to improve rates of osseous union. Autogenous iliac crest bone graft remains the gold standard biomaterial heralded for its biocompatibility and clinical success[23]; however, donor site morbidity and limited availability are disadvantages to this technique.[24]

Alternative harvest sites for cancellous graft have been identified. A popular strategy that can be used includes harvest from the femoral cavity using the Reamer-Irrigator-Aspirator technique (Fig. 3). A large quantity of autologous bone can be retrieved in minimally invasive fashion that qualitatively is superior to iliac crest bone graft in terms of the concentration of bone morphogenetic protein (BMP) and growth factors.[25,26]

With the advent of recombinant technology, highly concentrated BMP 2 and BMP 7 can be implanted at the site of tibial nonunion to hasten osseous union.[27] These manufactured growth factors can be combined with either autograft or allograft. Early clinical evidence has demonstrated that this methodology enhances osseous union when combined with cancellous autograft.[28] Further, BMP with allograft alone is comparable to autogenous grafting strategies.[29] Thus, donor site morbidity associated with autogenous graft retrieval is avoided. However, the use of recombinant BMP adds significant cost to the treatment plan.[30]

DISTAL TIBIA NONUNION WITH BONE LOSS

Bone loss in the metadiaphyseal region is not uncommonly associated with nonunion of the distal tibia. Addressing bone loss is an integral part of the plan of care. Bone defects typically occur in two different settings. First, bone loss can occur as a result of debridement of previously open fracture. Secondly, bone defect can occur as a result of debridement for previous infection.

A staged approach to the treatment of distal tibia nonunion in this setting is preferable. It is prudent to ensure that the site of nonunion is healthy and prepared to accept bone grafting procedure.[31] Without optimal conditions, success of bone grafting will be compromised as the biomaterial may not incorporate or, worse, serve as a septic nidus.

The first stage consists of debridement of the nonunion site to create a fresh osseous wound. All fibrous scar is removed. The bone is debrided

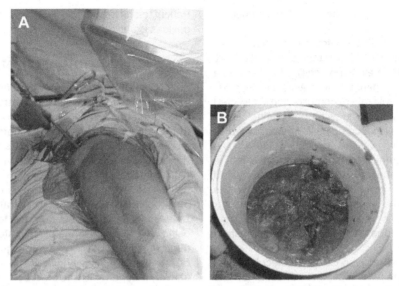

Fig. 3. As an alternative to iliac crest autograft, bone graft can be harvested from the femoral canal using the reamer-irrigator-aspirator method (*A, B*).

until healthy margins are realized. Furthermore, especially in cases of previous open fracture or infection, biopsy is retrieved to ensure that the nonunion site is aseptic.

Frequently, antibiotic beads will be placed to serve as a spacer for future bone graft procedure (**Fig. 4**). The beads will elute local antibiotics to the site of the nonunion to sterilize the wound bed; however, more importantly, the beads will incite an inflammatory response around the site

of bone loss. After a sufficient amount of time, a vascularized rind will form. This environment fosters the incorporation of bone graft applied during the final reconstructive stage.[32,33]

At the time of definitive reconstruction, the type of bone-grafting procedure performed is chosen based on the unique characteristics of the host and nonunion site. Autogenous bone graft procedure continues to be the gold standard method. However, availability of autogenous bone in each

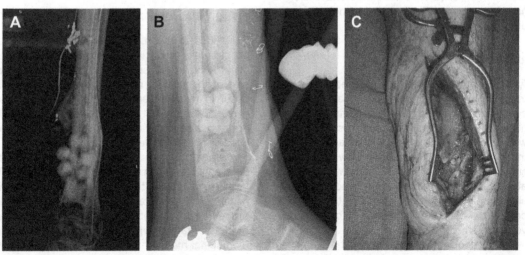

Fig. 4. Staged approach to infected distal tibia nonunion with bone loss. Previous exposed hardware removed, infected bone/soft tissue debrided, antibiotic beads placed, and free flap performed (*A, B*). After a course of organism-specific antibiotic therapy, definitive reconstruction performed using autogenous bone from the iliac crest and recombinant bone morphogenic protein (*C*).

particular case needs to be evaluated. Further, donor site morbidity must be weighed versus the inherent benefit for nonunion reconstruction.

With substantial bone defect, the bone graft can be used to serve two main purposes. The graft is the biologic scaffold to encourage osseous union across the nonunion site. Further, the graft can be used to enhance overall structural stability of the distal leg.

Structural grafts can be retrieved from the pelvis or the ipsilateral or contralateral fibula. Pelvic harvest is common either from the anterior or posterior iliac crest. Tricortical grafts can be retrieved with the precise geometry necessary to fill the area of bone loss providing both mechanical and biologic advantage to the site of nonunion.[34]

The fibula is also a popular graft for distal tibia nonunion and has been used in a variety of creative ways.[35–39] The fibula can be used as a biologic intramedullary implant. Depending on the location and size of the defect, a single- or double-barrel technique can be used. The fibula can be transferred as a nonvascularized graft or microvascular implantation is feasible. Further, the ipsilateral fibula adjacent to the nonunion site can be locally transferred with its adjacent soft tissue sleeve to serve as a biologic lateral plate.

Cancellous bone-grafting strategies either complement or are performed in lieu of structural grafts for the treatment of distal tibia nonunion. Cancellous grafts in an optimized soft tissue environment will serve as the ideal scaffold for osseous growth across bone defects. The pelvis and/or intramedullary canal of the femur are popular harvest sites. Bone grafts from these regions are heralded for their osteoconductive, osteoinductive, and sometimes osteogenic potential.

Cancellous bone graft can be placed directly into the bone defect site. However, the concept of central bone grafting has been popularized for nonunion of the distal tibia.[40] In addition to the placement of biomaterials at the site of nonunion, graft is placed along the anterior syndesmotic membrane. The goal is to create a distal synostosis by placing graft under the well-vascularized anterior compartment musculature.

Although autogenous bone grafting should be considered the gold standard treatment modality for distal tibia nonunion with bone loss, other innovative techniques are emerging. Bone graft extenders and osteoinductive agents are finding a prominent role in nonunion care. Their role is intended to reduce the donor site morbidity associated with autologous bone harvest. Further, the role of these biomaterials is critical when limited host availability of autogenous bone is a factor.

SUMMARY

A thoughtful treatment algorithm is required to optimally treat distal tibia nonunion. A healthy respect for the tenuous soft tissue envelope, compromised vascularity, and challenging mechanical environment is advisable. Achieving osseous union and improved functionality requires an individualized plan of care based on the personality of the nonunion and host. Attention must be focused on providing mechanical stability at the site of nonunion and providing biologic supplementation.

REFERENCES

1. Zelle BA, Bhandari M, Espiritu M, et al. Treatment of distal tibia fractures without articular involvement: a systematic review of 1125 fractures. J Orthop Trauma 2006;20(1):76–9.
2. Tarkin IS, Sop A, Pape HC. High-energy foot and ankle trauma: principles for formulating an individualized care plan. Foot Ankle Clin 2008;13(4): 705–23.
3. Attinger CE, Evans KK, Bulan E, et al. Angiosomes of the foot and ankle and clinical implications for limb salvage: reconstruction, incisions, and revascularization. Plast Reconstr Surg 2006;117(7 Suppl): 261S–93S.
4. Arany L, Baranyai T, Mândi A, et al. Arteriographic studies in delayed-union and non-union of fractures. Radiol Diagn (Berl) 1980;21(5):673–81.
5. Dickson K, Katzman S, Delgado E, et al. Delayed unions and nonunions of open tibial fractures. Correlation with arteriography results. Clin Orthop Relat Res 1994;302:189–93.
6. LeBus GF, Collinge C. Vascular abnormalities as assessed with CT angiography in high-energy tibial plafond fractures. J Orthop Trauma 2008;22(1): 16–22.
7. Borrelli J Jr, Prickett W, Song E, et al. Extraosseous blood supply of the tibia and the effects of different plating techniques: a human cadaveric study. J Orthop Trauma 2002;16(10):691–5.
8. Tarkin IS, Sojka JM. Biomechanical strategies for managing atrophic and oligotrophic nonunions. Operat Tech Orthop 2008;18(2):86–94.
9. Brinker MR, O'Connor DP, Monla YT, et al. Metabolic and endocrine abnormalities in patients with nonunions. J Orthop Trauma 2007;21(8):557–70.
10. Tarkin IS, Clare MP, Marcantonio A, et al. An update on the management of high-energy pilon fractures. Injury 2008;39(2):142–54.
11. Carpenter CA, Jupiter JB. Blade plate reconstruction of metaphyseal nonunion of the tibia. Clin Orthop Relat Res 1996;332:23–8.
12. Chin KR, Nagarkatti DG, Miranda MA, et al. Salvage of distal tibia metaphyseal nonunions with the

90 degrees cannulated blade plate. Clin Orthop Relat Res 2003;409:241–9.

13. Sheerin DV, Turen CH, Nascone JW. Reconstruction of distal tibia fractures using a posterolateral approach and a blade plate. J Orthop Trauma 2006;20(4):247–52.

14. Reed LK, Mormino MA. Distal tibia nonunions. Foot Ankle Clin 2008;13(4):725–35.

15. Reed LK, Mormino MA. Functional outcome after blade plate reconstruction of distal tibia metaphyseal nonunions: a study of 11 cases. J Orthop Trauma 2004;18(2):81–6.

16. DeOrio JK, Ware AW. Salvage technique for treatment of periplafond tibial fractures: the modified fibula-pro-tibia procedure. Foot Ankle Int 2003; 24(3):228–32.

17. Rijnberg WJ, van Linge B. Central grafting for persistent nonunion of the tibia. A lateral approach to the tibia, creating a central compartment. J Bone Joint Surg Br 1993;75(6):926–31.

18. Giannoudis PV, Pountos I, Morley J, et al. Growth factor release following femoral nailing. Bone 2008; 42(4):751–7.

19. Richmond J, Colleran K, Borens O, et al. Nonunions of the distal tibia treated by reamed intramedullary nailing. J Orthop Trauma 2004;18(9):603–10.

20. Abdel-Aal AM. Ilizarov bone transport for massive tibial bone defects. Orthopedics 2006;29(1):70–4.

21. Ring D, Jupiter JB, Gan BS, et al. Infected nonunion of the tibia. Clin Orthop Relat Res 1999;369:302–11.

22. Wukich DK, Belczyk RJ, Burns PR, et al. Complications encountered with circular ring fixation in persons with diabetes mellitus. Foot Ankle Int 2008;29(10):994–1000.

23. Meister K, Segal D, Whitelaw GP. The role of bone grafting in the treatment of delayed unions and nonunions of the tibia. Orthop Rev 1990;19(3): 260–71.

24. Mahendra A, Maclean AD. Available biological treatments for complex non-unions. Injury 2007;38(Suppl 4):S7–12.

25. Kobbe P, Tarkin IS, Frink M, et al. [Voluminous bone graft harvesting of the femoral marrow cavity for autologous transplantation. An indication for the "Reamer-Irrigator-Aspirator-" (RIA-) technique]. Unfallchirurgie 2008;111(6):469–72 [in German].

26. Kobbe P, Tarkin IS, Pape HC. Use of the "reamer irrigator aspirator" system for non-infected tibial nonunion after failed iliac crest grafting. Injury 2008; 39(7):796–800.

27. Johnson EE, Urist MR, Finerman GA. Distal metaphyseal tibial nonunion. Deformity and bone loss treated by open reduction, internal fixation, and human bone morphogenetic protein (hBMP). Clin Orthop Relat Res 1990;250:234–40.

28. Giannoudis PV, Kanakaris NK, Dimitriou R, et al. The synergistic effect of autograft and BMP-7 in the treatment of atrophic nonunions. Clin Orthop Relat Res 2009 [Epub ahead of print].

29. Jones AL, Bucholz RW, Bosse MJ, et al. BMP-2 Evaluation in Surgery for Tibial Trauma-Allograft (BESTT-ALL) Study Group. Recombinant human BMP-2 and allograft compared with autogenous bone graft for reconstruction of diaphyseal tibial fractures with cortical defects. A randomized, controlled trial. J Bone Joint Surg Am 2006;88(7):1431–41.

30. Dahabreh Z, Calori GM, Kanakaris NK, et al. A cost analysis of treatment of tibial fracture nonunion by bone grafting or bone morphogenetic protein-7. Int Orthop 2008 [Epub ahead of print].

31. Ristiniemi J, Lakovaara M, Flinkkilä T, et al. Staged method using antibiotic beads and subsequent autografting for large traumatic tibial bone loss: 22 of 23 fractures healed after 5–20 months. Acta Orthop 2007;78(4):520–7.

32. Pelissier P, Martin D, Baudet J, et al. Behaviour of cancellous bone graft placed in induced membranes. Br J Plast Surg. 2002;55(7):596–8.

33. Pelissier P, Masquelet AC, Bareille R, et al. Induced membranes secrete growth factors including vascular and osteoinductive factors and could stimulate bone regeneration. J Orthop Res 2004;22(1): 73–9.

34. Borrelli J Jr, Leduc S, Gregush R, et al. Tricortical bone grafts for treatment of malaligned tibias and fibulas. Clin Orthop Relat Res 2009;467(4):1056–63 [Epub 2009 Jan 15].

35. Ikeda K, Tomita K, Hashimoto F, et al. Long-term follow-up of vascularized bone grafts for the reconstruction of tibial nonunion: evaluation with computed tomographic scanning. J Trauma 1992; 32(6):693–7.

36. Chang MC, Lo WH, Chen CM, et al. Treatment of large skeletal defects in the lower extremities using double-strut, free vascularized fibular bone grafting. Orthopedics 1999;22(8):739–44.

37. Yajima H, Tamai S. Twin-barrelled vascularized fibular grafting to the pelvis and lower extremity. Clin Orthop Relat Res 1994;303:178–84.

38. Kassab M, Samaha C, Saillant G. Ipsilateral fibular transposition in tibial nonunion using Huntington procedure: a 12-year follow-up study. Injury 2003; 34(10):770–5.

39. Atkins RM, Madhavan P, Sudhakar J, et al. Ipsilateral vascularised fibular transport for massive defects of the tibia. J Bone Joint Surg Br 1999;81(6):1035–40.

40. Ryzewicz M, Morgan SJ, Linford E, et al. Central bone grafting for nonunion of fractures of the tibia: a retrospective series. J Bone Joint Surg Br 2009; 91(4):522–9.

Index

Note: Page numbers of article titles are in **boldface** type.

Orthop Clin N Am 41 (2010) 127–130
doi:10.1016/S0030-5898(09)00101-1
0030-5898/09/$ – see front matter © 2010 Elsevier Inc. All rights reserved.